Diabetic Yoga 1

M(

By:
Navneet Kaur

TABLE OF CONTENTS

LIST OF TABLES

LIST OF FIGURES

CHAPTER – I

INTRODUCTION

1.1 DIABETES AND GLOBAL SCENARIO

The occurrence of Diabetes is not only found in mid-age or older adults but it also affects the young population in the world (Guariguata et al., 2014). Globally, the prevalence of Diabetes Mellitus has been continuously rising and has become an epidemic. Approximately, 30 million individuals were earlier affected with Diabetes in 1964 (Entmacher and Marks, 1965).Ogurtsova et al. (2017) in their study showed that between the age group of 20-79 years, 415 million of the population was found battling with Diabetes causing a mortality rate of 5.0 million. Moreover, in 2015, the occurrence of Diabetes in adults was estimated at 8.8% and on the other hand, 16.2% of newborn had hyperglycemia (Ogurtsova et al., 2017). Due to increasing death rates until 2030, Diabetes Mellitus possibly became the 7th cause of death (Pal et al., 2017). Moreover, the International Diabetes Federation (IDF) has carried out the worldwide prevalence and estimation of this epidemic. The IDF shows the worldwide occurrence of Diabetes Mellitus viz. 151 million in 2000 [IDF, 1st edition, 2000], 194 million in 2003 [IDF, 2nd edition, 2003], 246 million in 2006 [IDF, 3rd edition, 2006], 285 million in 2009 [IDF, 4th edition, 2009], 366 million in 2011 [IDF, 5th edition, 2011], 382 million in 2013 [IDF, 6th edition, 2013] 415 million in 2015 (Ogurtsova et al., 2017), 451 million in 2017 (Cho et al., 2018). It was predicted by King et al., 1998 that in 2025 there will be 300 million adults diagnosed with Diabetes, 552 million in 2030 (Whiting et al, 2011), 592 million 2035 (Guariguata et al., 2014), 642 million in 2040 (Ogurtsova et al., 2017) 693 million in 2045 (Cho et al., 2018). Furthermore, it was revealed that individuals in low and middle-income countries record the greatest Diabetes incidence in the upcoming 22 years (Guariguata et al., 2014).

The incidence of Diabetes was more prevalent in the Western Pacific region (approximately 153.2 million) and Southeast Asia (56%) in 2015. Till 2040, the Middle East & North Region (103.8%) and African Region (140.7%) will witness maximum growth rates on a number of people with Diabetes (Ogurtsova, et al., 2017). Moreover, 48 % of the worldwide increase has been projected in India and China (Whiting et al., 2011). However, global expenditure due to this disorder was estimated

1

to be around 673 billion US dollars and likely to be increased up to 802 billion dollars in 2040 (Ogurtsova et al., 2017).

1.1.1 Diabetes and Indian scenario

The proportion of Diabetes is rapidly increasing not only worldwide but has also turned into a major health issue in India with an expected 66.8 million individuals suffering from this condition. In India, a large portion of health budget is spent on the treatment of Diabetes. Diabetes due to its increasing rate is found to deeply impact the economics of health spending. Therefore, it is imperative to improve the management, diagnostic and treatment strategies in the field (Joshi, 2015).

A survey conducted by Ramchandran et al. (2001), in six main cities, revealed that the occurrence of impaired glucose tolerance (IGT) and Diabetes was 14.0% and 12.1%respectively. This trend is more peculiar in urban India as compared to rural India (Ramchandran et al., 2001). India (31.7 million) is ranked first in the number of Diabetic cases in 2000 as compared with China (20.8 million) and USA (17.7 million) (Kaveeshwar and Cornwall, 2014). In India, 61.3 million people were identified with Diabetes in 2011, which is further expected to be projected to 101.2 million people by 2030 in India (Whiting et al., 2011). A study carried out by Indian Council of Medical Research (ICMR) shows the prevalence of Diabetes in four cities representing every region of India with 0.12 million people in Chandigarh, 0.96 million people in Jharkhand, 9.2 million people in Maharashtra and 4.8 million people in Tamilnadu (Anjana et al., 2011). Moreover, National Urban Survey, reported the prevalence of Diabetes in Northern India (Kashmir-6.1% and New Delhi-11.6 %), Western India (Mumbai-9.3 %), Eastern India (Kolkata-11.7 %) and Southern India (Chennai-13.5%, Hyderabad-16.6% and Banglore-12.4%) (Kaveeshwar and Cornwall, 2014). Moreover, in 2015 it was found that in India, 69.1 million individuals had second highest Diabetic cases after China (IDF, 7th edition, 2015).

In addition, many studies report that the occurrence of Diabetes Mellitus is increasing the financial burden among migrant Indians. The major causes are urbanization, changes in environment and lifestyle, abdominal obesity and genetic factors. Due to the Asian Indian phenotype and sedentary lifestyle, the visceral fat rises and high calorie and sugar diets make worsen among Indians have higher levels of insulin resistance and stronger genetic inheritance to Diabetes (Mohan, 2004).

2

Due to the rapid increase in Diabetes there are implications on health economics. Moreover, Grover et al. (2005) evaluated the economic burden on an individual, family and society due to Diabetes in their study. The result of the study revealed that the total yearly cost of care was Rs 14,508. The biggest extent of the aggregate cost comprises direct costs (68%), trailed by circuitous costs (28.76%) and supplier's costs (2.8%). The total treatment cost was altogether higher in the individuals who were more educated, the individuals who visited the hospital more regularly, and those consuming more drugs. They concluded in their study that Diabetes Mellitus is an expensive disease to treat even in developed countries.

According to ICMR-India DIABETES (2008-2011) study it has been estimated that incidences of Diabetes in urban areas is higher than the rural areas in Tamil Nadu (urban-13.7%, rural-7.8%), Jharkhand (urban-13.5%, rural-3%) Chandigarh (urban-14.2%, rural-8.3%) Maharashtra (urban-10.9%, rural-6.5%). However, in Chandigarh, the prevalence of Diabetes, both in urban as well as rural areas was higher than in comparison to the other three regions. They also showed in their report the prevalence of pre-diabetes in the four regions. In Tamil Nadu (urban-9.8% and rural-7.1%), Jharkhand (urban-10.7% & rural- 7.4%) and Maharashtra (urban-15.2% & rural-11.1%), the incidence of pre-diabetes is higher in urban areas, in comparison to rural areas, except Chandigarh (urban -14.5% & rural- 14.7%) where, the prevalence is slightly higher in rural areas in comparison to urban areas. Moreover, based on the Indian Diabetes Risk Score (IDRS) in Chandigarh-18.7%, Jharkhand-22.7%, Maharashtra-17.3% and Tamilnadu-27.6% subjects were found to have a high risk of developing Diabetes. The mean HbA1c (glycated haemoglobin) was highest in Chandigarh in both urban and rural areas (urban-8.7% and rural-9.3%) in comparison with the other three regions namely Tamil Nadu (urban-8.3% and rural-8.1%), Jharkhand (urban-8.2% and rural-8.3%) and Maharashtra (urban-8.0 and rural-7.9).

Nagarathna et al. (2020) performed the study on young adults, from 65 districts of India, among different age groups i.e. 19-22, 23-26, 27-30 and 31-34 years. The result of the study reported that number of Diabetic (22.36%) and pre-diabetic (9.86%) cases were more among 31-34 years of age group in comparison with other age groups. Moreover, those young adults who had Diabetic history of both the parents had more Diabetic (22.36%) and pre-diabetic (9.86%) cases in comparison with single

3

parent and no parent Diabetic history. The authors also demonstrated the positive correlation of HbA1c with BMI, family history of Diabetes and growing age.

Ravikumar et al. (2011), in their study, assessed the prevalence and risk factors associated with Diabetes in Chandigarh. Their community-based cross-sectional study from Chandigarh, for the age group of above 20 years, showed the occurrence of 11.1% and 13.2% for Diabetes and pre-diabetes respectively. They also showed the positive correlation between age, family history of Diabetes, obesity and hypertension with the presence of Diabetes.

1.2 DIABETES

Diabetes is a metabolic disorder that influences and alters carbohydrate metabolism, which further results in hyperglycemic conditions in blood. In the condition of hyperglycemia, there is an insufficiency of insulin production (Type 1 Diabetes) or inappropriate functioning of β-Cells of the pancreas (Type 2 Diabetes). There is an auto regulatory mechanism of our body in which upon food intake, the pancreas secretes an appropriate amount of insulin for transport of glucose into the cells. In conditions like Diabetes Mellitus, the pancreas makes a very small amount of insulin or no insulin. In certain cases, insulin resistance further results in the condition in which a large amount of glucose begins to rise in the blood. A continuous higher concentration of glucose in the blood leads to several metabolic alterations that result in various complications associated with Diabetes (American Diabetes Association (ADA), 2014).

1.2.1 History

"Diabetes" was named by the Greek physician, Aretaeus in 81-133AD on a Greek word "siphon" (Lakhtakia, 2013) at which he coined the term "the mysterious sickness" to describe Diabetes. The Mellitus word added by the "Dr. Thomas Wills", which means 'honey-sweet' to Diabetes after knowing the sweetness in both blood and urine in 1675. Furthermore, the occurrence of surplus glucose in blood and urine was recognized by the Dobson in 1776 (https://shodhganga.inflibnet.ac.in/bitstream/10603/62181/3/chapter-%202.pdf). Similarly, in 1921 the invention of insulin was done by doctors of Canada and they treated their patients of Diabetes with insulin to lower down the blood glucose levels (Ahmed, 2002). Many scientists and physicians from many years invented and innovated in the treatment of Diabetes.

4

1.2.2 Types of Diabetes Mellitus

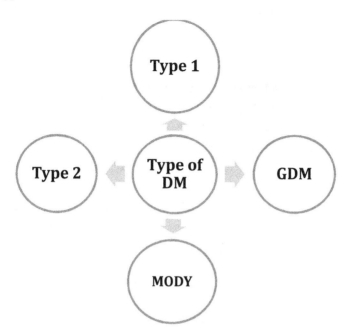

Figure 1.1: Schematic presentation of the various types of Diabetes Mellitus; **DM -** Diabetes Mellitus; **Type 1** -Type 1 Diabetes Mellitus; **Type-2** – Type 2Diabetes Mellitus; **GDM** – Gestational Diabetes Mellitus; **MODY** – Maturity onset Diabetes of young.

Type 1: Type 1 Diabetes (T1D) is a condition in which the pancreas secrete inadequate or no insulin, which is primarily caused due to theinefficiency of β-cells of the pancreas to secrete insulin (Ahmed and Goldstein, 2006). There are several molecular markers in the body that damage the immune pathways of β-cells including auto-antibodies to the tyrosine phosphatases (IA2 and IA-2 β), islet cells antibodies and autoantibodies to GAD (GAD65). T1D is closely linked with heredity and hereditary factors play a major role in damaging β-cells and environmental factors comparatively play a less important role in the onset of the disease. T1D contributes about 5-10% cases of all Diabetic cases (ADA, 2014)

Type 2: Type 2 Diabetes (T2D) is a prevalent form of Diabetes (Poulsen et al., 1999) which comprises of 90- 95% cases of all Diabetic cases (ADA, 2014). The main cause of T2D is dysfunctioning or deterioration of the regular functioning of pancreatic β-cells and insulin resistance (Ahmed and Goldstein, 2006), which leads to hyperglycemia in blood. The possibility of occurrence of T2D is mainly due to physical inactivity, age, heredity and excessive body weight.

Gestational Diabetes:

This form of Diabetes is characterized by its occurrence at the time of pregnancy. The worldwide prevalence of Gestational Diabetes is approximately 7.0% while in Asian region it varies from 0.7 % to 51.0 % (Lee et al., 2018). In this form of Diabetes, a woman develops a condition of glucose intolerance that is first detected during pregnancy (Landon et al., 2009). Women who had a parental history of Diabetes and excessive body weight develop a higher risk for the development of gestational Diabetes (Lavery et al., 2017). Moreover, Gestational Diabetes increases the risk of T2D in mother and their offspring in the near future (Lee et al., 2018).

Maturity onset Diabetes of Young (MODY):

This type of Diabetes is very rare and follows a very strong genetic pattern and is also related with hyperglycaemia and transmitted as autosomal dominant trait in the individual younger than 25 year (ADA, 2010).

1.2.3   Symptoms of Diabetes:

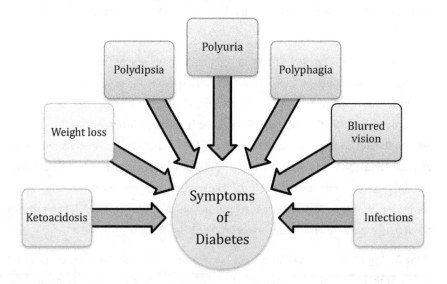

Figure 1.2: Symptoms related to Diabetes (ADA, 2014)

Symptoms:

➢ **Ketoacidosis:** It is a condition in which the body produces excess body acids due to non-production of insulin in the body. Moreover, symptoms like vomiting, nausea, thirst, polyuria, weakness, abdominal pain are noticed.

➢ **Weight loss:** Individuals with Diabetes are not able to utilize the calories present in the food, even though they consume a sufficient amount of food. For instance, sugar and water losses in the urine and develop dehydrating conditions in the body and results in weight loss.

➢ **Polydypsia (Extreme Thirst):** The situation of Polydypsia occurs in the condition of hyperglycemia. To maintain normal glycemic conditions, the body requires more water to compensate for high blood glucose, which is replenished, by the water during the polyuria.

➢ **Polyuria (Extreme Urination):** To get rid of hyperglycaemic conditions the body tries to eliminate excess glucose from the blood by excreting it through urine, which further leads to dehydration by extreme water loss.

➢ **Polyphagia (Extreme eating):** In T2D, insulin resistance stimulates hunger in the body and due to insulin resistance, the level of insulin is increased in the body resulting in increased appetite.

➢ **Infections:** Occurrence of various types of infections i.e. genital infection, skin infection, urinary tract infections are very common in hyperglycaemic individuals because of poor functioning of the immune system and bad blood glucose control.

➢ **Blurred vision:** Due to the high amount of blood glucose the vision gets blurred and it may further leads blindness (Ministry of AYUSH, 2017, https://antidiabetesayush.wordpress.com/2017/05/25/yoga-protocol-for-control -of-diabetes/).

1.2.4 Risk factors promoting Diabetes

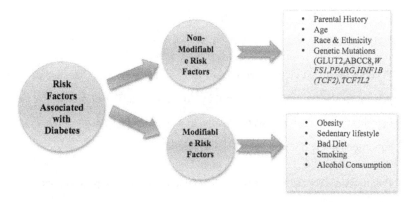

Figure 1.3: Representation of various risk factors associated with Diabetes.

The various risk factors associated with Diabetes include:

Non-modifiable risk factors:

Parental History:

The family history of the individual is one of the major non-modifiable risk factors, which results in a propensity for Diabetes. Those people who have a family history of Diabetes are 50% more vulnerable to Diabetes in comparison with a non-Diabetic family history (Abate and Chandila, 2001). Moreover, recommendations from the ADA (2007) suggest screening for Diabetes for those whose first-degree relatives (a mother, father, sister, or brother) are Diabetic.

Age:

The risk of T2D is increased with growing age. The prevalence of Diabetes has increased from 2.0% (20-44 years) to 18.7 % (65-74 years) (Harris et al., 2000). There is evidence to show that middle and older aged individuals are at a greater risk for onset of Diabetes Mellitus especially people with age of 45-64 years at utmost risk for development of disease (Shantakumari et al., 2013).

Race and Ethnicity:

It is widely believed that race and ethnicity are also linked with the prevalence of Diabetes in specific ethnic populations namely African Americans, Mexican Americans, American Indians, native Hawaiians and some Asian Americans. This

8

could be because of varying incidences of hypertension, Diabetes and obesity in these ethnic groups. While African Americans have greater chances for the onset of Diabetes in comparison with other ethnic groups (Boulton et al, 2005) whereas among Asian Indians poor glucose control is linked with early incidence of Diabetes (Vijayakumar et al., 2017).

Modifiable risk factors:

Diet:

An unhealthy diet and irregular eating pattern leads to health-related problems for the individual. A population-based cross-sectional survey (NFHS-3, 2005-2006) carried out in all states of India aimed to know the prevalence of Diabetes at all India level. They reported that the prevalence of Diabetes differs from region to region, southern, northern and eastern zone report a higher risk of Diabetes in comparison with the rest of India. They further reported in their study that intake of fruits, pulses and beans moderate disease prevention (Agrawal and Ebrahim, 2012).

Obesity:

Obesity is a modifiable risk factor for developing T2D(Gillet et al., 2012). For instance, obesity also promotes insulin resistance in the body, which is due to the over-production of adipokines by adipose tissue (Kahn et al., 2006). The data from two national surveys revealed that the risk of Diabetes escalates with increased body mass index (BMI) (Bays et al., 2007)

Alcohol consumption:

The intake of alcohol correlates with poor blood glucose control in Diabetes. Continuous alcohol consumption brings unfavourable impact on the liver (Ben et al., 1991). A meta-analysis by Huang et al. (2017) has shown that individuals with higher alcohol consumption had a higher risk of Diabetes in comparison with individuals with moderate alcohol consumption. This is up to 30 % less than in comparison with high-risk individuals.

Smoking: Some studies have shown the correlation of smoking with an increased risk of T2D in an individual (Willi et al., 2007). The data in the study also demonstrates the effect of smoking on insulin sensitivity, pancreatic β cell functioning and body

9

composition (Stadler et al., 2014). Smoking and nicotine exposure also affects glucose homeostasis (Tweed et al., 2012).

Stress: Stress also plays a major role in the pathophysiology of Diabetes (Detka et al., 2013) In stressful conditions, the sympathoadrenal system and Hypothalmic Pituitary Adrenal (HPA) (Smith and Vale, 2006) get activated which results in catecholamine release, cortisol secretion resulting in various pro-inflammatory cytokines which leads to insulin resistance and T2D.

Lack of physical activity: In the modern world, individuals follow a sedentary lifestyle, which leads to many lifestyle-related disorders. Lack of physical activity results in the increased risk of Diabetes and its associated comorbidities. It has also been shown in a study that people who prefer physical workout than a sedentary lifestyle have 3 times less Diabetic risk than physically active people (Mohan et al., 2003).

1.2.5 Complications:

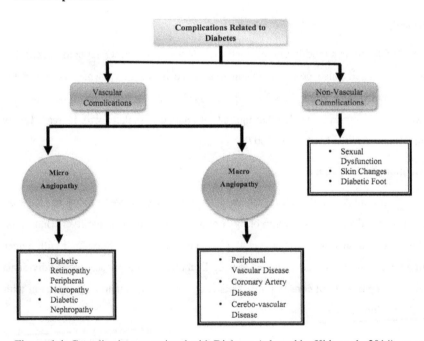

Figure 1.4: Complications associated with Diabetes (adapted by Kide et al., 2014)

Complications:

Diabetes Mellitus is a serious chronic disorder, which leads to many complications and health risks in afflicted individuals. Complications associated with Diabetes affect various organs and systems in the body, which eventually result in mortality, disability, and a decrease in Quality of Life (QoL). Diabetes also causes damage to various blood vessels, which can be either macro-angiopathy (large blood vessel disease) and micro-angiopathy (small Blood vessel disease). Micro angiopathy includes complications of retinopathy, peripheral neuropathy and Diabetic nephropathy (Gartner and Eigentler, 2008). In retinopathy, macular edema causes severe loss of vision and even blindness. Additionally, peripheral neuropathy occurs in a combination of damaged blood vessels and result in foot ulcers and increases the progression to necrosis, gangrene, amputations of limb and infections. Diabetic Nephropathy causes end-stage renal failure and impairment of glomerular filtration (Alsaad, 2007).

In macro angiopathy complications, Peripheral Vascular Disease (PVD), Coronary Artery Disease and Cerebrovascular Disease occur. PVD is associated with Diabetic patients and is characterized by complications related to vascular muscle cell dysfunction, inflammation, endothelial dysfunction are the main causes in Diabetic arteriopathy(Huysman and Mathieu, 2009)

Diabetes Mellitus is closely associated with cardiovascular diseases (CVD) and coronary heart disease. CVD contributes to 65 to 75 percent of deaths among Diabetic patients (Ali et al., 2010). Furthermore, Diabetic people have 2-4 times greater risk for onset of coronary disease and they are 2 to 6 times vulnerable to Stroke (Ergul et al., 2012). Diabetes exerts adverse effects on every part of the body, which includes skin, feet, eyes and sexual dysfunction (Aalto, 1997).

1.2.6   Diagnosis:

The timely screening of the individuals needs to be carried out to understand the Diabetic status of the individual. There are following tests for the diagnosis of Diabetes.

11

Fasting Blood Glucose (FBG):

Fasting blood glucose is measured when an individual has not eaten or taken a drink for at least 8-10 hours. There is a specific range of the FBG for categorization into normal (<100), pre-diabetes (100-125) and Diabetes (>125) (ADA, 2010).

Oral glucose tolerance test (OGTT):

The Oral glucose tolerance test (OGTT) measures the blood glucose level in an individual after 8 hours of fasting and then the individual is given glucose (75 gm) beverage and after 2 hours, the sample is taken again for measurement. If a person exhibits values greater than or equal to 200 mg/dl, he/she is considered as Diabetic (ADA, 2010).

Glycated Haemoglobin (HbA1c):

HbA1c is used as a gold standard for diagnosing Diabetics and preDiabetics. American Diabetes Association suggests HbA1c test to estimate the glycemic index of an individual. The range of normal, PreDiabetic and Diabetic is <5.7, 5.7-6.4 and >6.5 respectively (ADA, 2010).

1.2.7   Treatment:

The pharmacological treatments of Diabetes include insulin. Endocrinologists also refer to oral anti Diabetic drugs (OAD) like thiazolidinedione, alpha-glucosidase inhibitors, etc. (Pal et al., 2017). For the treatment of Diabetes, OADs were used which provides relief to the patients but there are also side effects of these pharmacological treatments such as diarrhea, Nausea, Vomiting and Gastric problems (Bastaki, 2005 and Pal et al., 2017). The accumulation of Diabetes Mellitus may be delays by adoption of lifestyle modifications tools with the intake of different combinations of drug metformin, acarbose, voglibose and troglitazone (Ramchandran et al., 2006 and Chiasson et al., 2002).

1.2.8   Management of Diabetes Mellitus:

The report published by WHO recommends promotion of healthy habits like healthy food habits (less consumption of fast food), reduced or nil tobacco intake (through smoking, chewing, etc.), regular physical activity to maintain normal body weight and continuous monitoring for early screening of Diabetes associated retinopathy, neuropathy and kidney disease (Centers for Disease Control and Prevention, 2014).

1.3   PRE-DIABETES

Pre-diabetes is an intermediate condition between normal glycemic and hyperglycaemic levels in the blood. It is defined as borderline differentiation between Diabetes and normal individuals. The pre-diabetic individuals show higher glucose level greater than the normal individual but lesser than the Diabetic individuals (Ferrannini et al., 2011). Pre-diabetic individuals have higher susceptibility to develop T2D. Every year, 5–10% of people with pre-diabetes develop Diabetes and convert back to normal. The incidence of pre-diabetes is rising globally with the projection of 470 million individuals who may have pre-diabetes by 2030. The pre-diabetic condition has arisen due to β-cell dysfunctioning and insulin resistance. Pre-diabetes is also linked with the early stages of various complications associated with Diabetes viz. Diabetic retinopathy, Diabetic nephropathy, blurred vision, peripheral neuropathy, and Diabetic foot. The lifestyle modification tools play a significant role in the life of pre-diabetic individuals by preventing the onset of Diabetes Mellitus in individuals with a 40-70% decrease in the risk level (Tabak et al., 2012).

The pre-diabetes is an indicator of IGT condition, which is reflected as a measure of blood glucose level [postprandial blood glucose (PPBG)] and fall into the range of 140 to 199 mg/dl as per applicable guidelines. Another parameter impaired fasting glucose (IFG) which is measured through the level of blood glucose before taking a meal is referred to as FBG and required as a clinical biomarker which establishes a criteria for screening of pre-diabetes if an individual's blood glucose values fall within the range of 100 to 125 mg/dl.

For screening of pre-diabetic individuals among the community, both the methods i.e FBG & PPBG are considered (International Expert Committee, 2009). But there are some chances of error in the results based upon FBG and PPBG values. Hence, there was a need for exploring new effective biomarkers that validate the results based on glucose level and provide insights about mechanisms. In 2010, ADA,

13

recommended the use of HbA1c for the screening of pre-diabetes if it falls between 5.7 to 6.4 percent. HbA1c is another potent marker along with IFG/FBG for the screening of pre-diabetic population. Time period of transition of pre-diabetes to Diabetes is quite long but it is rarely found to be an early onset of the transition with a transition rate of 70 percent if not proper monitoring or careless approach in early stages of pre-diabetes were taken (Markin and Micheal, 2011).

1.3.1   The scenario of Pre-diabetes

The global prevalence of pre-diabetes has been accelerating each day. The global occurrence of pre-diabetes among adult population (20-79 years) is 352.1 million in 2017, which will be expected to increase upto 587 million in 2045. In addition, maximum number of population (72.3%) resides in low and middle income countries (IDF, 8th edition, 2017 and Alrefai et al., 2019). The maximum worldwide prevalence of Impaired Glucose tolerance was found in North America and Caribeban (15.4%) followed by Central and South America (10.0%), Europe (5.5%), South East Asia (3.0%) respectively (IDF, 8th edition, 2017 and Hostalek, 2019).

According to the National Urban Diabetes Survey, they projected the occurrence of 14% pre-diabetes in the Indian population (Ramchandran et al., 2001). They also reported in their survey done in 6 major cities that out of 6 major cities 4 cities had shown a higher occurrence of IGT than T2D. The maximum prevalence of IGT found in Chennai (16.8%) followed by Bengaluru (14.9%), Hyderabad (29.8%), Kolkata (10%), Mumbai (10.8%), and New Delhi (8.6%) respectively. According to another survey carried out by the Indian Council of Medical Research-India Diabetes, it was predicted that there was a prevalence of 62.4 and 77.2 million Diabetic and PreDiabetic individuals respectively in the Indian Population. The estimated percentage of pre-diabetes in Tamilnadu, Maharashtra, Jharkhand and Chandigarh were 8.3%, 12.8%, 8.1% and 14.6% respectively (Anjana et al., 2011). Moreover, it was also found in a study that Asian Indians develop more rapidly to Diabetic stage from pre-diabetic stage than another ethnic population (Anjana et al., 2015 and Sattar and Gill, 2015)

1.3.2 Pathophysiology of Pre-diabetes

Pre-diabetes is initial or early-stage for progression to the Diabetes. Pathophysiology of pre-diabetes is characterized by increased levels of insulin resistance and inefficiency of insulin secretion (Rhee & Woo, 2011). In preDiabetic condition, the fasting plasma insulin is found increased. The insulin resistance is seen in various tissues of the body like liver, muscle and fatty cells. People with IGT, have hepatic insulin resistance (in postprandial condition), which is indicated by impaired hepatic glucose production (HGP) by insulin. Moreover, the IGT individuals have hepatic insulin resistance but the level of insulin resistance is reduced in comparison with people with IFG (Ghani et al., 2006). People with IGT have elevated levels of fasting plasma free fatty acid (FFA) concentration, which is due to Adipocytes. Adipocytes are inhibited by insulin. Due to increased plasma FFA concentrations, it results in insulin resistance in skeletal muscle in IGT people (Ghani and DeFrenzo, 2009). Adipocytes insulin resistance is seen in both IFG and IGT individuals. There is a direct linkage between the severity of insulin resistance and the degree of glucose tolerance (https://shodhganga.inflibnet.ac.in/bitstream/10603/14118/8/08_chapter%201.pdf.)

Pre-diabetic individuals experience that the increase in insulin resistance is interlinked with several metabolic defects like obesity, dyslipidemia and hypertension, they are major contributing risk factors for CVD (Defronzo, 1997 and Reaven, 1988) regardless of the presence of normal glucose levels (Cersosimo and Defronzo, 2006).The incidence of metabolic abnormalities is enhanced 2-3 folds in pre-diabetics as compared to normal individuals (Alexander et al., 2003).

1.3.3 Insulin Secretion in Pre-diabetes

In the physiology of insulin secretion, the main path of glucose uptake is through Gasteronintestinal Tract by triggering the production of Incretin hormones i.e glucagon-like peptide 1 (GLP-I) and gastric inhibitory peptide (GIP), which activates the secretion of insulin by acting upon β, cell. Incretin hormones are those hormones that stimulate insulin production in response to the meal uptake. In pre-diabetic condition (IFG and IGT) intensity of insulin secretion is seen dysregulated in β-cell functioning (Ferrannini et al., 2005). In addition, the decrease in the rate of GLP-1 or resistance to GIP in preDiabetics may lead to a decline in β-cell sensitivity to glucose

15

and dysregulated insulin secretion (Ghani and Defronzo, 2009). However, insulin resistance was more progressive initially in the individuals those had parental history of T2D along with continuous β-cell failure, which is considered as one of the key factors in the accumulation of T2D (https://shodhganga.inflibnet.ac.in/bitstream/ 10603/14118/8/08_chapter%201.pdf.)

1.3.4 Treatment of Pre-diabetes

Various worldwide organizations viz; Health Services in India (IHS), Diabetic Association (DA) and American Association of Clinical Endocrinologists (AACE), Canadian Diabetes Association (CDA) and Australian Diabetes Society (ADS) recommends treatment of pre-diabetes. Some Organizations i.e AACE and ADA recommend a treatment regime for halting the conversion of pre-diabetes to Diabetes. The ADA and AACE recommend lifestyle modifications along with metformin (ADA, 2011) and some other organizations i.e IHS, CDA and ADS highly recommend usage of oral anti-Diabetes drug like (thiazolidinedione, alpha glucosidase inhibitor, etc.). Moreover, they also advocate the utility of modification in lifestyle as a preventive approach for managing and reducing pre-diabetes and delay the onset of Diabetes (Ramchandran et al., 2006; Chaisson et al., 2002 and Twigg et al., 2007). The main advantage of lifestyle modification tools is that it had no side effects whereas oral antiDiabetic drugs had shown some side effects like gastritis, hypoglycemia, vomiting and nausea etc.

Various changes at the physiological and cellular level result into impaired insulin secretion and resistance (Kanat et al., 2011), which continues into mild inflammation that leads to conversion from pre-diabetes to Diabetes (Grossmannm et al., 2015). In pre-diabetic condition, micro and macrovascular complications began to arise (Tabak et al., 2012) along with cardiovascular complications (Giraldez et al., 2013).

1.3.5 Diagnostic Criteria for Pre-diabetes

- Fasting Blood Glucose (FBG), 100 – 124 mg/dl (Ministry of AYUSH, 2017)

- Post Prandial Blood Glucose (PPBG),140-199 mg/dl (Ministry of AYUSH, 2017)

- Glycated Haemoglobin (HbA1c), 5.7-6.4% (ADA, 2010)

16

1.3.6 Major risk factor for Pre-diabetes

- Family History of Diabetes
- Sedentary Lifestyle/ Lack of Physical activity
- Race/Ethnicity
- Abdominal/Central Obesity
- Body mass index ≥ 25 kg/m^2
- History of gestational Diabetes
- Women suffered from polycystic ovarian syndrome

1.3.7 Management of Pre-diabetes:

Pre-diabetic is a condition in which an individual is at high risk for onset of T2D along with cardiovascular diseases. So, it is imperative to prevent and delay the conversion of pre-diabetes to Diabetes at the early stages(Matfin and Pratley, 2010). Lifestyle modification tools are one of the most effective non-pharmacological ways for the management of pre-diabetes and the prevention of Diabetes and the various risk associated with it. Implementation of regular physical exercise regime in the lifestyle helps pre-diabetic individuals. For instance, GLUT4, which is insulin responding glucose transporter, improves insulin sensitivity and peripheral glucose uptake at the surface of the cell by regular physical activity (Ferrari et al., 2019). Moreover, Hordern et al. (2012) reported in their study that exercise has shown a beneficial impact on optimum glycemic control and preventing the progression of T2D. They further recommend vigorous-intensity exercise and moderate-intensity exercise for 125 and 210 minutes per week respectively. Moreover, excessive body weight plays a prominent role in the onset of T2D. Abdominal obesity is among one of the modifiable risk factors for the onset of T2D (Bjorntorp, 1988). A study by Wing et al. (2011) revealed that reduction of weight up to 4.5 kg decreases the risk of T2D by ~ 30%.

1.4 INDIAN DIABETES RISK SCORE (IDRS): THE RISK STATUS FOR DIABETES

Indian Diabetes risk score (IDRS) is a non-pharmacological method for risk analysis. IDRS is very easy to use and cost-effective method to know the risk of Diabetes among the community. This tool is constructed by Mohan et al. (2005)from

17

their cohort Chennai urban rural epidemiology study (CURES). IDRS is based on four risk factors; two modifiable (physical activity and waist circumference) and two non-modifiable (age and family history) risk factors. These risk factors are closely associated with CVD and metabolic syndrome. The final IDRS score was obtained by adding the score for each factor. Through IDRS one can check his or her level of risk of Diabetes and can timely take proper preventive measures.

1.5   YOGA

Yoga according to MahrishiPatanjali mentioned in Patanjali Yoga *Sutra* 1st chapter and second sutra is:

$$योगश्चित्तवृत्तिनिरोधः ॥२॥$$

Yogash-chitta-vritti-nirodhah ||2||

Yoga is defined as a state in which one's controls their mind and thoughts (Devi, 2010) in which *vrittis*(delusion) occurs in the changeable attributes of the individuals *(chitta)* vanished (https://www.ashtangayoga.info/philosophy/source-texts-and-mantra/yoga-sutra/chapter-1/)

Yoga is ancient traditional knowledge and believed to be discovered 5000 years ago, which focuses on the overall well being of the individual i.e physical, mental and spiritual. The word Yoga is derived from the sanskrit word '*Yuj*' which means 'to unite one's body, soul and mind'. Hence, Yoga is the unification of body, mind and soul with supreme power *(Parmatman)*. Many people have argued that Yoga is also another type of physical activity that involves twisting, turning, stretching and breathing in the rhythmic and synchronized manner. However, these are only the superficial aspects of yogic science, which gradually progresses from simple loosening exercises to complex *asanas*, and *pranayama,* which stimulate various '*Kundalies*' inside the human body. A detailed and analytical study by Khalsa et al. (2007) revealed the promising potentials of Yoga for serving mankind. In the modern scenario, Yoga is getting popular day by day due to its possible benefits in preventing the onset of various diseases and their related complications. Yoga is one of the cost-effective (Bali et al., 2020) and non-pharmacological ways of adopting a healthy lifestyle. In the modern world, there is a huge amount spent on health budget due to the rise in various types of diseases and complications but by focusing on the preventive aspect of a disease one can reduce the cost spent on the cure of the diseases. In addition, many studies recommended the role of Yoga in the amelioration of pre-diabetes and Diabetes in an effective way.

1.5.1 *Ashtanga*Yoga: A way of life

Maharishi Patanjali is considered as the father of Yoga. MaharishiPatanjali is the founder of *Ashtang* Yoga and one can able to control his mind through practice of *Ashtanga* Yoga. Maharishi Patanjali mentioned about *Ashtanga*Yoga in Pantanjali Yoga *sutras* 2nd chapter and 29th*sutras* is:

yamaniyama-asana pranayama pratyaharadharanadhyanasamadhayo-'shtavangani ||29||

यमनियमाअसनप्राणायामप्रत्याहारधारणाध्यानसमाधयोऽष्टावङ्गानि॥२९॥(*https://www.as*

htangayoga.info/philosophy/source-texts-and-mantra/yoga-sutra/chapter-2/)

"*Ashtanga* Yoga is defined as the process of sublimation of all mental modifications in the mind through a systematic process of *Yamas* (moral doctrines), *niyamas*(disciplines), *asanas* (postures), *pranayam* (regulated nostril breathing), *pratayhara* (drawing the mind away from perceptible external sensory stimuli), *dharana* (concentration) *dhyana* (meditation) and *Samadhi* (absorption)" (Rao et al., 2017). The main goal of Yoga is to develop self-awareness which is achieved through eight limbs of Yoga (Garfinkel and Schumacher, 2000).

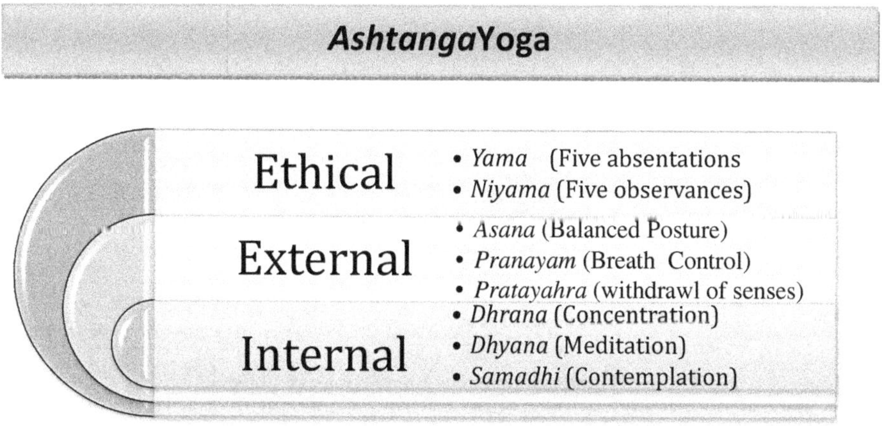

AshtangaYoga

Ethical	• *Yama* (Five absentations • *Niyama* (Five observances)
External	• *Asana* (Balanced Posture) • *Pranayam* (Breath Control) • *Pratayahra* (withdrawl of senses)
Internal	• *Dhrana* (Concentration) • *Dhyana* (Meditation) • *Samadhi* (Contemplation)

Figure 1. 5 : *Ashtanga* Yoga

19

1.5.2 Diabetic Yoga Protocol (DYP):

Diabetic Yoga Protocol (DYP) is the first ever standardized Yoga protocol developed by committee of 16 experts through Delphi protocol discussions chaired by Dr. H.R Nagendra specifically for pre-diabetics and fit Diabetics who can perform the practices. DYP is approved by Government of India. The total duration of DYP is of 60 minutes comprising of 30 minutes to physical activity another 30 minutes assign to pranayama and relaxation. DYP is starts and closes with prayer (Ministry of AYUSH,https://antidiabetesayush.wordpress.com/2017/05/25/yoga-protocol-for-control-of-diabetes/)

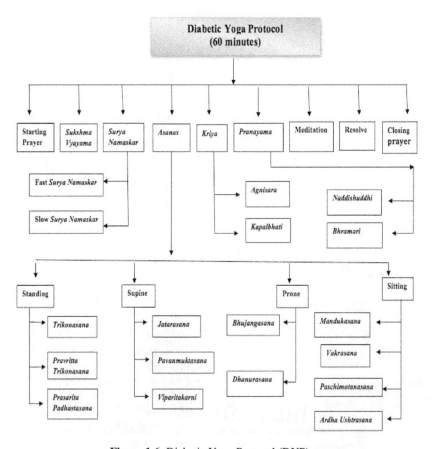

Figure 1.6: Diabetic Yoga Protocol (DYP)

20

1.   Opening Prayer:

DYP is started with prayer with both hands joining in *Namaskara Mudra*.

ॐअसतोमासद्गमय।

तमसोमाज्योतिर्गमय।

मृत्योर्माअमृतंगमय।

ॐशान्तिःशान्तिःशान्तिः ॥

Om AsatoMaa Sad-Gamaya |

TamasoMaaJyotir-Gamaya |

Mrtyor-MaaAmrtamGamaya |

Om ShaantihShaantihShaantih ‖

The meaning of this prayer is:

"Is to take from ignorance lead me to truth; from darkness, lead me light; from death, lead me to immortality; *Om* peace peacepeace".

2.   Loosening Exercises (*SithilikaranaVyayama*) and *Suryanamaskara*

In this protocol, in the beginning the opening prayer *SithilikaranaVyayama* was rendered. *SithilikaranaVyayama* is performed with breathing and awareness. The loosening exercises include simple trunk movements, which result in bringing the flexibility to the body. Loosening exercises prepares the body for *suryanamaskara*. Loosening exercises start with slower rhythmic movements, which gradually become faster. The rhythmic movements coupled with breathing pattern bring deep internal awareness to the part where stretch feels during particular *asanas*. It provides warmth to the body, loosening of muscles, suppleness and elasticity of the body, which prepares body for risk free Yoga practice.

After loosening exercises, *suryanamskara* was performed which is intermediate between loosening exercise and *asanas*. *Suryanamaskara* is a set of 12 postures, which was in the beginning done with fast movements and then done slowly. For instance, in fast *suryanamakara* the calories all over the body are burnt and slow *suryanamaskara* brings deep awareness in the body. The rhythmic blend of breathing and body movements helps in enhancement of concentration and body awareness.

Apart from this, the chair *suryanamskara* was included in the protocol, for person with medical reasons and other physical problems (Ministry of AYUSH,https://antidiabetesayush.wordpress.com/2017/05/25/yoga-protocol-for-control-of-diabetes/).

Asanas:

Suryanamsaka is followed by set of *asanas*. *Yogasanas* is defined as *"SthiraSukhamAsanam"* which meansto maintain the final posture for long time with comfort and further it becomes easy, effortless and joyful. In this protocol, the *asanas*are divided into their different positions like standing (*trikonasana, pravarittatrikonasana, prasarittapadotanasana*), supine (*jataraparavaritasana, pavanmuktasana, vipratkarani*), prone (*bhujangasana, dhanurasana, pawanmuktasana*) and sitting (*mandukasansa, pachimotanasa, vakrasana/ ardhmatsayndrasana, ardhaustrasana*).

Asanas helps in conserving the energy; it works in synchronization with nature. It is the stretch with awareness and gradually slowing down with the aim of self mastery through asanas that helps cells to perform better. Regular practice of asana result into conscious, wakeful relaxation to the nervous system, musculoskeletal system and endocrine system (Ministry of AYUSH, https://antidiabetesayush. wordpress.com/2017/05/25/yoga-protocol-for-control-of-diabetes/).

Pranayama:

Pranayam is made up of two words. *Prana* and *Ayama*. *Prana* means a pranic energy, which accounts for life force to carry out overall functions of the body. *Ayama* means to control. In other words, we can say that *pranayama* means to control over breathing or achieve mastery over *prana*. Intially, *prana* drawn from the base of the spine and reach to all parts of the body through *nadis* and *chakras*. Every cell in the body needs *prana* to perform their functions efficiently. *Pranayama* helps in awakening of inner spritiual force and bring calmness to the mind. Moreover, the sickness in the body is due to uncontrolled excessive *prana* during stress, due to increased speed of mind the excess *prana* causes imbalance in the nadis disrupting healthy functioning of the chemical processes in the tissues, damge/inflammation in the tissue. Therefore, for reducing the flow of *prana* the locked *prana* from injured organ achieved by cleansing breathing practices like *kapalbhati* and slow breathing practices *(pranayama)e.g.* breathing at the rate of 1-2 breath per minute. By practice of slow breathing *pranayama* one can achieve the mastery over excessive speed of *prana*. There are many types of *pranayama*, which includes fast breathing, slow breathing, alternate nostril breathing, Uni-nostril breathing, each type of breathing related with mastery over prana and correct the imbalances related with them. In this protocol, *agnisarakriya* and one cleansing technique with inclusive *kapalbhati.Nadhishudhhi* and *bhramari pranayama* are included for balancing of *prana* (Ministry of AYUSH, https://antidiabetesayush.wordpress.com/2017/05/25/ yoga-protocol-for-control-of-diabetes/).

Meditation:

Meditation is uninterrupted, flow of mind towards the specific object. Meditation is known to bring awareness, which makes definite changes in cognition, attention and perception. The processes of meditation follows specific pattern viz; single thought effortlessness, awareness, calmness and expansiveness. The practice of meditation is believed to decrease sympathetic activity, breath rate and anxiety. Furthermore, it improves cardiac vagal activity, attention and concentration. In addition, it generates hypo metabolic physiological state with maximum control over mind, which further helps in controlling of Diabetes (Ministry of AYUSH, https://antidiabetesayush.wordpress.com/2017/05/25/yoga-protocol-for-control-of-diabetes/).

Resolve:

Meditation is followed by resolve in which one speaks to himself and reassures 'I am Happy'.... 'I am Healthy'

Closing Prayer:

The Protocol ends with closing prayer:

ॐसर्वेभवन्तुसुखिनः।
सर्वसन्तुनिरामयाः।
सर्वेभद्राणिपश्यन्तु।
माकश्चित्दुःखभाग्भवेत्॥
ॐशान्तिःशान्तिःशान्तिः॥

Om SarveBhavantuSukhinah

SarveSantuNiraamayaah |

SarveBhadraanniPashyantu

MaaKashcid-Duhkha-Bhaag-Bhavet |

Om ShaantihShaantihShaantih ||

The meaning of this prayer 'Let all be happy, free from diseases. Let all align with reality, let no-one suffer from miseries' (Ministry of Ayush, 2017).

Om Peace Peace Peace.

Each and every step of Yoga enhances the physical strength, endurance, empowers mind, brings emotional stability and enlightens the soul. The regular practice of Yoga benefits promotion of health, prevention and management of diseases and mental disturbances and to attain the higher level of consciousness.

1.5.3 Yoga and Diabetes

Exercise and Yoga are believed to exert long term glycemic control. Glycemic index and glucose levels could be maintained through change in life style and food habits. However, reduction in weight, optimal glucose levels and wellness can be achieved by regular Yogic practices. Yoga comprises of various physical and respiratory exercise, therefore, it can be a suitable integral therapy for Diabetic patients mediated by improvement of musculoskeletal and cardiopulmonary function and also by improves mental health (Vizcaino and Stover, 2016).

Recently, Diabetes can be developed irrespective of age, place or heredity. However, the condition can be regulated with increased community awareness and care at pre-diabetic level. Moreover, by doing a regular Yoga practice, a person can be empowered to regulate the glucose level through mind-body harmonization. Yogic practices can be effectively used as the preventive care treatment in pre-diabetic individuals. There are many such studies that found the significant effect of Yoga in human physiology.

The effects of aerobic exercises and Yoga on Diabetics have demonstrated safe and significant results (Cai et al., 2016). Meta-analysis has shown that yogic practices can provide homeostasis by maintaining various biochemical factors that indicate blood profiling (fasting glucose, haemoglobin, total cholesterol, high density lipoprotein, low density lipoprotein and triglyceride etc.) that suggest the its beneficial effects on Diabetes Mellitus patients. (Cui et al., 2016). Moreover, Rajesh et al. (2013) have also reported significant decrease in blood sugar levels and improved cardiac function after one month Yoga practice in age group of 30-60 years old participants. Similar study was carried out on Diabetic patients in order to analyze the effect of same duration Yoga intervention with age range of 35-60 years. Authors have found that one month Yogic practices can help in reducing the plasma glucose levels in Diabetic patients (Vinutha, et al., 2015).

Lately, Santhakumari et al. (2016) have shown the effect of yogic practices on memory due to glycosylation of haemoglobin in Diabetic patients. However, the levels of N-Acetyl Aspartate (NAA) and Myoionositol (mI) in right and left frontal lobe did not show any difference in both the groups, but overall memory in Diabetic patients was increased among the individuals who practice Yoga.

Moreover (Sahay, 1986) revealed in their study that practice of *Pranayama* brings reduction on the intake of insulin and oral glycemic agents along with significant decline on the values of insulin glucose ratio, FBG & PPBG.

25

Another study done on Non-insulin dependent Diabetes Mellitus (NIDDM) participants (30-60 years) demonstrated significant results of 40 days Yoga Practice (30-40 min/Daily) on glycemic parameters i.e. FBG, PPBG, HbA1c and oxidative stress (Singh et al., 2001).

Additionally, Yoga *asanas* brings significant reduction on the insulin levels and waist hip ratio. Yoga practice also helpful in utilization of glucose, which further support the fact that Yoga might be used as adjuvant therapy for amelioration of T2D along with drugs and diet (Malhotra et al., 2005).

Furthermore, in another study Yoga based lifestyle change program demonstrated the significant decline on Fasting **B**lood Sugar (FBS), HbA1c, lipid profile, insulin resistance, psychological parameters (anxiety & depression) and increased in QoL (Nagarathan et al., 2008). Further, the scholar try to fill the research gap that majority of the above mentioned studies do not describe attendance based variation in various biochemical or clinical changes as quality assurance is lacking.

1.6   LIFESTYLE MODIFICATION TOOLS

In modern scenario, there is a unhealthy lifestyle pattern followed by the people which includes luxuries lifestyle, bad eating habits (consumption of fast food), sedentary lifestyle, irregular sleeping pattern etc. Lifestyle modification tactics mainly focused upon the promotion of regular physical activity and inclusion of healthy and balanced diet in the lifestyle, which is, recommends by the clinicians for prevention and management of pre-diabetes and Diabetes (Tuomilehto et al., 2001; Knowler et al., 2002; Li et al., 2008 and Perreault et al., 2012). Various study done in different countries reported the postive effects of life style modification programmes on prevention and management of Diabetes (Lindstrom et al., 2006; Knowler et al., 2002; Ramchandaran et al., 2007; Tuomilehto et al., 2001 and Li et al., 2001). Hence, lifestyle modification tools considered as best effective way for preventing the conversion from pre-diabetes to Diabetes (Tuomilehto et al., 2001).

1.7   WOMEN AND DIABETES

Diabetes Mellitus is one of the leading chronic epidemic worldwide. Particularly, in women the relationship among coronary heart disease and Diabetes more prevalent among females than males (Castelli, 1988) upto 50 % more in females

26

(Huxley et al., 2006) which is mainly due to the reason that women might be having more prominent cardiovascular risk (Wingard et al., 1995 and Fuller et al., 1979). Moreover, in comparison with male, female had higher levels of blood pressure and lipids, (Huxley et al., 2006) the mortality risk was higher among females then in males when coupled with coronary risk and Diabetes which is might be due to lack of receiving of standard treatment (Huxley et al., 2006).

The study done by Hu et al., 2001 conducted a 16 years follow up and found that BMI is the prominent risk factor for T2D. The women with BMI 35 or above had comparative risk of 38.8; BMI with 30.0 to 34.9 had risk of 20.1, in comparison with BMI less than 23.0. The normal range BMI with end (23.0 to 24.9) less than 23.0 (relative risk, 2.67). Furthermore, physical inactivity was directly associated with Diabetes for e.g. the comparative risk for women who had been exposed to physical activity for seven or more hours per week in comparison with those had completed physical activity for less than half an hour was 0.48 (Hu et al., 2001). Even women who don't have Diabetes have the risk of development of gestational Diabetes during their pregnancy. Moreover, Polycystic Ovary Syndrome (PCOD) is also known to be associated with Diabetes risk primarily due to insulin resistance, which is more pronounced in PCOD. In addition, women suffered from Diabetes also battling with problems like depression, stress and sexual health (Centers for Disease Control and Prevention, 2018).

Kautzky et al. (2016) reported in their study that the T2D is more often in men with lower age and BMI while in women obesity is more prevalent which is a major risk factor for Diabetes. There are various risk factors which affect includes genetic, nutritional and inactive lifestyle besides biological and psychosocial factors that are applicable in both genders. In addition, sex hormones have a major effect on body composition, vascular function and inflammatory responses. The hormonal imbalances like excess of androgens in women and hypogonadism in men are associated with unfavourable cardiometabolic traits. Women are more affected with stress in comparison with males. Gestational Diabetes needs special care in view of the health of offsprings.

In India, a study on T2D women explored bicultural perspective. The authors analyzed, in a set of 280 females without diabetes, and those with T2D women for health, social roles, biological correlations, and their inter-relationships that prevail between Diabetes, social role attainment, psychological stress, and biochemical variables assessing blood sugar control, immune stress, and generalized inflammation. The level of blood sugar and HbA1c has shown poor management in women. This is due to changing immune stress, which often accompanies uncontrolled blood sugar (Weaver et al., 2015).

Due to our cultural and social constraints, women give preference to their domestic roles rather than their own health. This results in poor Diabetes control at the expense for others. A lady is generally perceived as a sacrificial figure, which at times represents a conflict between culture and health (Weaver et al., 2015).

Moreover, women's continuous ignorance of their health results in poor mental health due to perform their social roles. Specifically in North India, a patriarchal society makes it unfeasible for women to prioritize their own health. Women with Diabetes have generally poor Diabetic control associated with increased inflammation, immune stress, depression, poor mental health and physical disability. A study suggests that Diabetes care guidelines could be positioned in such a way so as to promote the idea that women are made aware of the need to care for themselves (Weaver et al., 2015). Promotion of health among women indirectly promotes the health of a family. Therefore, it is a necessary for women to maintain good health, mental peace and a balanced life. Yoga can be an effective method to address health complications arising in post modern scenario (Mudliar, 2013).

1.8 ANGIOGENESIS, APOPTOSIS, NEUROGENESIS, STRESS AND COGNITIVE IMPAIRMENT IN DIABETIC PATHOLOGY

Expression pattern of vascular endothelial growth factor (VEGF) and BCL-1 can provide molecular insights of effect of Yogic practices on angiogenesis and apoptosis. VEGF hypomethylation has revealed that pre-eclampsia can be regulated by VEGF and its associated receptors (Sundrani et al., 2013). Similarly, analysis of methylation of VEGF promoter and its regulatory proteins can open a new vista for therapy of cancer and age-related macular degenaration (AMD) pathobiology (Kim et

28

al., 2012). 12 week exercise program to obese elderly women can reduce the VEGF levels and also help in maintaining the structure and function of carotid artery, further signifying the effective regulation of lipid metabolism and VEGF mediated pathways (Park et al., 2010). Moreover, decreased expression of VEGF in pancreatic β-cells can hamper the effectiveness of insulin and consequently lead to the pre-diabetic condition in adults. Similarly, systematic review on effect of exercise on the VEGF expression has been done in elderly persons. The results have demonstrated the increased expression of VEGF in these populations (Vital et al., 2014). Therefore, studies have suggested the stimulatory or pro-angiogenic effect of exercise/Yoga of angiogenesis and its impact on overall well being can be useful in health promotion.

Diabetes is one of the causes for various complications associated with brain functions including cognitive decline and depression. Various studies have examined the negative impact on neurogenesis, dendritic remodelling and increased apoptosis of the neuronal cells in the Diabetic condition. Pathological changes in hippocampal region induced with Diabetic condition leads to various brain related complications, which involves in learning, memory and emotional expression (Ho et al., 2013).

Study conducted byBathina et al. (2017) suggests that impaired memory, learning, and cognitive dysfunction witnessed in persons with Diabetes Mellitus could be because of Brain-Derived Neurotrophic Factor (BDNF) deficiency. Similarly, Ortiz et al. (2016) have examined the relationship ofBDNF with cognitive impairment in patients with T2D. Their study revealed that the levels of BDNF showed considerable variations between patients with T2D (43.78 ± 9.05 vs 31.55 ± 10.24, $P = 0.005$), like low levels of BDNF are coupled with cognitive impairment in patients with T2D.

Neuhauer et al. (2016) studied angiogenin level in middle-aged T1D patients and concluded that in spite of the presence of Diabetic microangiopathy, angiogenin level in middle-aged T1D patients is lower than the control subjects without Diabetes. The angiogenin level in patients with overt Diabetic nephropathy was higher when compared to patients without nephropathy. However, Chiarelli et al. (2002) focused on serum angiogenin concentrations in young patients with Diabetes Mellitus. Their study revealed that angiogenin serum concentrations are increased in Diabetic children even before puberty and young patients with microvascular complications

29

have significantly high angiogenin levels. Long-term tight glycemic control shows a consistent lessening of angiogenin concentrations. Moreover, Dworacka et al. (2015) demonstrated that Alpha-Lipoic Acid (ALA) may affect angiogenesis in type 2 Diabetic patients through an impact on some circulating factors including VEGF, Basic Fibroblast Growth Factor (bFGF), Monocyte Chemoattractant Protein-1 (MCP-1) and Interleukin 10 (IL-10). The findings in their study revealed that ALA notably increased VEGF, bFGF and IL-10 and decreased MCP-1 serum concentrations in patients with T2D with coronary artery disease (CAD) and Diabetic Distal Sensorimotor Polyneuropathy (DSPN). Whether these alterations vary among ayurgenotypes after Yoga intervention has not been investigated.

Previous studies supports the role of leptin in case of insulin secretion (Tanizawa et al., 1997), which is associated with Diabetes Mellitus. The available evidence indicates that leptin exerts inhibitory efforts on pancreatic β-cell. Leptin, which is produced by adipo tissues, and insulin, is known to stimulate adipogensis in these tissues. According to Seufart et al. (1999), insulin stimulates leptin secretion &leptin inhibits insulin, production β-cell because of dysregulation of a adipoinsular axis (Seufert et al., 1999). Stress is one the major concern in women health and predominantly occurs in girls, housewives as well as in working women too. Cortisol levels were found to be higher in the Diabetic pathology and it also depends on the duration of Diabetes, sex and HbA1c. Results show enhanced HPA activity in Diabetic patients (Chiodini et al., 2007). Diabetic pathology has been found to be associated with various complications. The Yogic practices can boost women health by regulating the various cellular mechanisms and their associated biomolecules.

Yoga can also play an important role in reversal of pathological condition raised due to altered expression of above said molecules. But there are a few studies on Yoga and their effect on homeostasis that regulates the various mechanisms mediated through these proteins. Therefore, the present study can pave way in the treatment and management of pre-diabetic condition and its associated complications through Yogic practices.

RATIONALE OF THE STUDY

Diabetes is a metabolic disorder, which is not treatable after its onset, but it can be controlled by early detection of the high risk individuals. It will be useful to halt the onset of Diabetes, either mediated by various molecular or epigenetic changes through Yoga, which is a non-pharmacological approach method. This can act as the transforming agent for pre-diabetic individuals to become normal. In the present study, we have attempted to study the role of DYP in biochemical and molecular profile of pre-diabetic women and also map the attendance based variations in the selected biochemical and molecular profile used in the present study among pre-diabetic women.

STATEMENT OF THE PROBLEM

The problem is entitled as **"Role of Diabetic Yoga Protocol in Biochemical and Molecular Profile of Pre-diabetic Women"**

AIM OF THE STUDY

To investigate the effect of Diabetic Yoga protocol on biochemical and molecular profile of pre-diabetic women.

OBJECTIVES OF THE STUDY

1. To examine the effects of DYP on Biochemical variables i.e. FBG and HbA1c among pre-diabetic women.

2. To examine the effects of DYP on Anthropometric variables viz. Weight, BMI, Waist circumference (WC), Hip Circumference (HC) and Waist Hip Ratio (WHR) among pre-diabetic women.

3. To examine the effects of DYP on Neuropsychological variables i.e. State anxiety, Perceived stress, Sustained attention and General health among pre-diabetic women.

4. To examine the effects of DYP on Molecular markers viz. Angiogenin, VEGF and BDNF among pre-diabetic women.

31

5. To examine the effects of DYP on Hormonal Markers i.eLeptin and Cortisol among pre-diabetic women.

6. To examine the effects of DYP on overall Quality of Life (QoL) and its domains among pre-diabetic women.

7. To examine the effects of practicing DYP for 6 weeks and 12 weeks on Biochemical variables viz. FBG and HbA1c among pre-diabetic women.

8. To examine the effects of practicing DYP for 6 weeks and 12 weeks on the selected Anthropometric variables i.e. Weight, BMI, WC, HC and WHR among pre-diabetic women.

9. To examine the effects of practicing DYP for 6 weeks and 12 weeks on selected Neuropsychological variables i.e. State anxiety, Perceived stress, Sustained attention and General health among pre-diabetic women.

10. To examine the effects of practicing DYP for 6 weeks and 12 weeks on Molecular markers viz. Angiogenin, VEGF and BDNF among pre-diabetic women.

11. To examine the effects of practicing DYP for 6 weeks and 12 weeks on Hormonal Markers i.eLeptin and Cortisol among pre-diabetic women.

12. To examine the effects of practicing DYP for 6 weeks and 12 weeks on overall Quality of life (QoL) and it's associated domains among pre-diabetic women.

HYPOTHESIS OF THE STUDY

1. There would be significant effects of DYP practice on selected Biochemical variables i.e FBG and HbA1c among pre-diabetic women.

2. There would be significant effects of DYP practice on selected Anthropometric variables viz. Weight, BMI, WC, HC and WHR among pre-diabetic women

3. There would be significant effects of DYP practice on selected Neuropsychological variables i.e. State anxiety, Perceived stress, Sustained attention and General health among pre-diabetic women

4. There would be significant effects of DYP practice on selected Molecular Markers viz. Angiogenin, VEGF and BDNF among pre-diabetic women.

5.   There would be significant effects of DYP practice on selected Hormonal markers i.e. Leptin and Cortisol among pre-diabetic women

6.   There would be significant effects of DYP practice on overall QoL and its associated domains among pre-diabetic women.

7.   There would be significant effects of practicing DYP for 6 week and 12 week on selected Biochemical variables viz. FBG and HbA1c among pre-diabetic women.

8.   There would be significant effects of practicing DYP for 6 week and 12 week on selected Anthropometric variables i.e. Weight, BMI, WC, HC and WHR among pre-diabetic women.

9.   There would be significant effects of practicing DYP for 6 week and 12 week on selected Neuro-psychological variables i.e. State anxiety, Perceived stress, Sustained attention and General health among pre-diabetic women.

10.   There would be significant effects of practicing DYP for 6 week and 12 week on Molecular markers viz. Angiogenin, VEGF and BDNF among pre-diabetic women.

11.   There would be significant effects of practicing DYP for 6 week and 12 week on Hormonal markers i.e. Leptin and Cortisol among pre-diabetic women.

12.   There would be significant effects of practicing DYP for 6 week and 12 week on total QoL and its domains among pre-diabetic women.

DELIMITATIONS OF THE STUDY

1.   The present study was delimited to female subjects only.

2.   The participants aged between 20 to 70 years were recruited.

3.   The present study was delimited to selected rural and urban area residents of Chandigarh only.

4.   Only with consent of pre-diabetic women with IDRS ≥ 60 were recruited in the present study.

5.   Yoga protocol for Diabetes control developed by Ministry of AYUSH, India was administered.

LIMITATIONS OF THE STUDY

1. Diabetic patients were not included in the present study.

2. Pre-diabetic women who have undergone any kind of surgery were excluded from the present study.

3. Pre-diabetic women having history of head injury, psychiatric disorder, severe cardiac disease, were excluded from the present study.

4. Any bias in the subject's response to the questionnaire was not in control of researcher.

5. Further, the education and socio-economic status of selected subjects were out of control of the researcher.

6. During the days of application of training protocol, the aptitude of the subjects might have been influenced the result of the present study.

7. The present study was conducted for over a span of twelve weeks; the variations in the environmental conditions and the level of acclimatization were beyond the control of the researcher.

8. All outside activities, food habits, social habits of the participants were not in the control of the researcher.

9. No specific motivational technique was used during the training protocol.

DEFINITIONS OF THE OPERATIONAL TERMS

YOGA

"Yoga is an ancient art based on a harmonizing system of development for the body, mind and soul"(Trivedi and Raval, 2016).

PRE-DIABETES

"Pre-diabetes, defined by blood glucose levels between normal and Diabetic levels" (Edwards and Cusi, 2016).

Tabla 1.1. Diabetes Diagnostic Criteria (ADA, 2010 and Ministry of AYUSH, 2017)

Sr.No	Diabetes diagnostic test	Normal	Pre-diabetes	Diabetes Mellitus (DM)	Units of measurement
1	Glycated haemoglobin (Hb1Ac)	< 5.7	5.7-6.4	≥ 6.5	Percent
2	Impaired Fasting Glucose (IFG)/ FBG	80- 100	100 – 124	≥ 125	mg/dl
3	Impaired Glucose tolerance (IGT)/ PPBG	< 140	140-199	≥ 200	mg/dl

DIABETIC YOGA PROTOCOL (DYP)

'Diabetic Yoga Protocol' consists of standardised sequence of *asanas, pranyama* and meditative practices specifically for pre-diabetics made by committee of experts constituted by Ministry of AYUSH. In the present study 'Diabetic Yoga Protocol' was administered on experimental group (high risk women).

GENERAL HEALTH

"Health is defined as a state of complete physical, mental, and social well-being and not merely the absence of disease or infirmity" (WHO, 2006). In the present study 'General Health' was measured by the General Health Questionnaire-12 (GHQ-12) by Goldberg et al., 1997.

QUALITY OF LIFE (QoL)

"It is defined as individual's perceptions of their position in life in the context of the culture and value systems in which they live and in relation to their goals, expectations, standards and concerns" (Vahedi, 1997). In the present study the Quality of Life (QoL) was measured by the WHOQOL-BREF scale constructed by World health Organization, 2004.

PERCEIVED STRESS

"It refers to an individual's perceived response to interaction with his or her environment" (Cohen et.al, 1983). In the present study perceived stress was measured by Perceived Stress Scale (PSS) developed by Cohen et al., 1994.

SUSTAINED ATTENTION

Sustained attention is the ability of an individual to perform the task within specific time, which further shows the individual focus and mental stability. In the present study the sustained attention was measured by six letter cancellation test (SLCT) by Natu and Agarwal, 1997.

STATE ANXIETY

"State anxiety reflects the psychological and physiological transient reactions directly related to adverse situations in a specific moment" (Leal et al., 2017). In the present study state anxiety was measured by using the sub scale of State-trait anxiety inventory by Spielberger (1983, 2010).

ANGIOGENESIS

"Angiogenesis is the generation of new blood vessels from pre-existing ones" (Tahergorabi and Khazaei, 2012).

VEGF

Vascular endothelial growth factor (VEGF) is involved in angiogenesis. In the present study, VEGF protein was seen in blood serum and estimated by ELISA.

ANGIOGENIN

It is a protein which involved in angiogenesis processes. In the present study, Angiogenin protein was seen in blood serum and estimated by ELISA.

NEUROGENESIS

"Neurogenesis, is a process of generating functional neurons from neural precursors" (Ming and Song, 2011).

36

BDNF

Brain-derived neurotrophic factor (BDNF)is a protein, which is involved in neurogenesis. In the present study, BDNF protein was seen in blood serum and estimated by ELISA.

LEPTIN

It is a hormone formed by adipocytes, which controls the balance of energy by suppressing hunger. In the present study, Leptin was seen in blood serum and estimated by ELISA.

CORTISOL

It is a hormone, which released in response to a stress. In the present study, Cortisol was seen in blood serum and estimated by ELISA.

BLOOD GLUCOSE

The concentration of glucose (sugar) in blood measured in mmol/L or mg/dl. In the present study, blood glucose was estimated in diagnostic laboratory after blood collection.

GLYCATED HAEMOGLOBIN (HbA1c)

"HbA1c monitors the exposure to circulating glycaemia in the previous 3 months" (Tavares et al., 2016). In the present study, glycatedhaemoglobin was estimated in diagnostic laboratory after blood collection.

SIGNIFICANCE OF THE STUDY

The present study investigates the preventive effect of Diabetic Yoga Protocol in pre-diabetic individuals along with their wellness, mediated by various molecules, which are known to play a crucial role in health management. The present experimental study provides a mechanism that links the molecular and cognitive effects arising from practice of Diabetic Yoga protocol. This type of study has never been undertaken describing the effect of standardized Diabetic Yoga Protocol, examined at molecular and cognitive level. The results might prove useful in establishing the integration of Yoga with the modern medicine.

Further, the present study establishes a link between cognitive, ayurgenomic and molecular changes resulting from Yoga intervention in pre-diabetic individuals. The present study can generate the evidence whether that Yoga practices can bring overall homeostatic changes in the pre-diabetic women.

The study can provide the insights for lifestyle disorders like Diabetes, associated behaviour and stress related complications and their management through Yogic practices, specifically in women. The findings of the study will not only add to the knowledge of Psychologists, Educationists, Physical Educationists, Counsellors, Clinicians and General public but also enable them in effective handling of Diabetes Mellitus by encouraging pre-diabetic victims to adopt a healthy lifestyle through Yoga therapy.

The present study can also proves helpful in managing co-morbidities related with the Diabetes i.e. various cardiac disorders, stroke, Diabetic nephropathy, Diabetic retinopathy, Diabetic foot, peripheral neuropathy etc. Further, in reference to health expenditure or health cost, the prevention and management of Diabetes Mellitus through Yogic interventions involve negligible investment and superior outcomes which not only reduce the economical burden on an individual and their family but also helpful in reducing the economical burden of the nation.

CHAPTER –II
REVIEW OF RELATED LITERATURE

Adhikari et al. (2010) conducted a study for validation of Indian Diabetes Risk Score (IDRS) in coastal population of Karnataka. For the purpose of the study 551 volunteers were enrolled in the study. The OGTT was performed on the participants after intake of 75 gram glucose. Authors reported in their study that, among the study participants the number of people with known Diabetic and newly Diabetic were 71 and 45 respectively. They further concluded that IDRS is an efficient tool for screening and risk detection of high risk individuals for Diabetes in the community.

Anjana et al. (2011) has revealed that except Tamilnadu the Diabetes patients exceed the ratios of 1:1 in all regions. The general occurrences of pre-diabetes in Tamilnadu, Maharashtra, Jharkhand and Chandigarh was8.3%, 12.8%, 8.1% and 14.6% respectively. There are almost 0.12 million and 0.13 million people affected with Diabetes and pre-diabetes respectively in Chandigarh. The study has also estimated that people in India most probably converted to Diabetes (around 62.4 million) and pre-diabetes (around 77.2 million).

Cahn et al. (2017) explored the effect of 3-month Yoga and meditation on 38 healthy individuals. The assessments were carried out at baseline (pre-test) and after 3 months for BDNF, psychological parameters, pro-inflammatory and anti inflammatory markers. The result of the study revealed that Yoga and meditation practice shows reduction in anxiety and depression whereas improvements on Brain Derived Neurotropic Factor (BDNF) and cortisol awakening response were also concurred. Furthermore, the Interleukin-10 (IL-10) (anti- inflammatory markers) was increased and Interleukin-12 (IL-12) (pro-inflammatory marker) was decreased. The study also emphasized that enhanced BDNF levels were seen as a possible moderator for health.

Chimkode et al. (2015) studied on subjects (36-55 Years) with Diabetes (minimum 1 Year duration and on Diabetic diet and anti Diabetic drugs) and without Diabetes to understand the effect of 6 month regular Yoga practices on glycemic parameters i.e.

Fasting Blood Sugar (FBS) and Post Prandial Blood Sugar (PPBS). The assessment was taken at 3 and 6 months. After 6 months, FBS and PPBS showed decline in both the Yoga groups. However, after three months of Yogic practices significant decline was observed for selected variables in Type 2 Diabetes (T2D) group in comparison to the control group.

Cotman et al. (2007) it has been examined that exercise enhances the synaptic plasticity by directly influencing the synaptic structure and potentiating synaptic strength, and by strengthening the underlying frameworks. Moreover, growth and genesis could be regulated by insulin growth factor-1 (IGF-1), BDNF and Vascular Endothelial Growth Factor (VEGF) which can be induced by exercise that directly support that neurogenesis, learning, and angiogenesis can be modulated with the effect of exercise .

Datey et al. (2018) conducted a study on pre-diabetic male prisoners with elevated FBS and PPBS. The authors evaluated the impact of 3 month Yoga practices along with administration of fresh herbal juices on blood glucose and HbA1c levels. The subjects were divided into three groups viz. *Rasahara* + Yoga, Yoga alone and control (no intervention) group. The result of the study showed significant decline in FBS and PPBS levels in *Rasahara* + Yoga group and FBS level in Yoga group. However, control group witnesses the increase in the PPBS levels.

Gordon et al. (2009) showed the effects of 24 weeks *Hatha* Yoga and physical training exercise programmes on biochemical variables, oxidative stress markers and oxidant status in patients with T2D. The study comprises of three groups i.e. *Hatha* Yoga group, physical training exercise group and control group. Biochemical and oxidative stress markers studied at baseline and 3 months showed significant reduction in the levels of FBS ($P < 0.0001$) serum total cholesterol ($P < 0.0001$) very low density lipoprotein ($P = 0.036$ in both Hath Yoga and physical exercise group after 3 months. Moreover, Malondialdehyde ($P < 0.0001$) significantly decrease while the activity of superoxide dismutase significantly increased ($P = 0.031$). This study suggested the preventive effect of *Hatha* Yoga exercise and conventional physical training exercise on Diabetes Mellitus.

Gustafsson et al. (1999) analysed the mRNA expression of VEGF, fibroblast growth factor (FGF-2) and hypoxia induced factor (HIF) in exercised group. The expression of VEGF and HIF-1α were found to positively correlate with exercise in human skeletal muscle.

Halappa et al. (2018) stated in their study that 12 weeks Yoga practices contributes in significant improvement in BDNF concentrations and neuropsychological test performance in comparison to the controls in depressive patients. The authors further reported in their study that Yoga + medicines or Yoga alone are promising approach for bringing positive changes on neuroplaticity and neuropsycological functioning in depressive patients.

Hegde et al. (2011) aimed to investigate the comparative effect of 3 months Yoga practices + standard care group and standard care alone group on anthropometrical profile, glycemic profile, oxidative stress and blood pressure in patients with T2D. The findings of the study shows that significant decline was seen on BMI, glycemic parameters, malondialdehyde whereas rise in glutathione and vitamin C was seen in Yoga practices + standard care group in comparison to the standard alone care group. However, for blood pressure, waist circumference, WHR, vitamin E and superoxide dismutase no significant changes were seen in Yoga practices + standard care group. This study further supports the efficacy of Yoga in regulation of oxidative stress.

Jagannathan et al. (2015) investigated the occurrence of T2D among Yoga practitioners in two districts from south (Ernakulam) and east (Pune) India. The assessments included FBS and Diabetes risk assessment. The overall occurrence of Diabetes in Yoga practitioners at Pune and Ernakulam was 3.6 % and 26 % respectively. The overall percentage for Diabetes "at risk" among Yoga practitioners at Pune and Ernakulam District was 18.9 % and 12 % respectively. Among Yoga practitioners, growing age and short term Yoga practice was strongly associated with the elevated risk of Diabetes. The authors concluded in their study that for better management of Diabetes the individual need to done regular checkups for Diabetes after the 40 years of age and also need to engage in lifestyle modification tools i.e. Yoga for longer duration.

41

Jyotsna et al. (2012) explored the impact of Yogic breathing practices (*Sudarshan Kriya* Yoga + *pranayama*) along with anti-diabetic drugs on Diabetic patients who had HbA1c between the range of 6-9%. The patients were divided into two groups viz. one group received Diabetes standard treatment alone and another group received Diabetes standard treatment + Yogic breathing practice for 6 months. The assessments for various glycemic parameters (FBS, PPBS & HbA1c) and Quality of Life (QoL) were done for 6 months. The findings of the study shows that Yogic breathing practices + standard treatment group had better control on glycemic parameters than Diabetes standard treatment alone group but not at significant level. However, overall QoL was significantly increased in Yogic breathing practices + standard treatment group in comparison with Diabetes standard treatment only group.

Kacker et al. (2019) explored the impact of three months Yoga interventions in prediabetic subjects (N= 102) on lipid and glycemic parameters. The subjects were segregated into equal groups, Yoga (n= 51) and control group (n= 51). The study highlights the significant decrease in glycemic (blood glucose & HbA1c) and lipid parameters (cholesterol, triglyceride and low-density lipoprotein) in Yoga group when compared with control group. This study further suggest the beneficial impact of Yogic practices in controlling glycemic and lipid parameters in pre-diabetic subjects.

Kaur et al. (2020) had done a case report to investigate the impact of Yoga on Obesity. The authors reported significant reduction in Body Mass Index (BMI) in the case. The assessment for BMI was taken at baseline (33.2 kg/m^2), one month of yoga practice (31.1 kg/m^2) and after two months (29.4 kg/m^2). Kaur et al. (2020) state that obesity is one of the risk factor for the Diabetes and by ameliorating obesity it further helps in better risk management of Diabetes.

Keerthi et al. (2017) aimed to study the impact of 12 weeks Yoga practices on IDRS and QoL in normotensive young adults with Diabetes and pre-diabetes. They comparedin their study the effect of standard treatment alone group with combination of standard treatment and Yoga group among Diabetic and pre-diabetic subjects. The significant difference in QoL and IDRS was observed when combination of standard treatment & Yoga was given in comparison to when there was standard treatment alone.

42

Kiecolt et al. (2012) examined the effects of *Hatha* Yoga on stress reduction. They compared naive and experts in Yoga on adiponectin and leptin level. The results of the study showed that level of leptin was higher among Yoga novices in comparison with experts. However, the adiponectin levels were higher in Yoga practitioners in comparison to naive.

Kontoangelos et al. (2015) explained the relationship of homocytesine and cortisol with psychological factors in T2D. The result of the study revealed that the connection between psychoticism and homocyteine is positive within controlled Diabetic patients they also showed significant relationship between homocysteine and act-out hostility scale. They further concluded in their study that homocysteine and cortisol are associated with trait and state psychological factors in patients with T2D.

Kraus et al. (2004) revealed that skeletal muscle capillary supply is an essential determinant of maximum exercise capacity which is regulated by VEGF. VEGF is formed by skeletal muscle cells and can be secreted into the circulation. The authors studied the difference between well-trained endurance athletes and sedentary individuals on circulating VEGF levels in response to acute exercise as well as at rest. Eight male endurance athletes and sedentary subjects was taken in the study and they performed the exercise (50% of maximum power output) for 1 hour. The plasma was collected from the subjects at 0, 2 and 4 hour after the exercise for estimation of plasma VEGF levels. The result of the study revealed that after 0 and 2 hour of the exercise VEGF levels were significantly increased in endurance athletes. However, in sedentary subjects no increase in plasma VEGF levels was seen at any point of time. Further, in reference to different time point, no significant difference was observed between endurance athletes and sedentary subjects on VEGF levels. Although, the rise in VEGF levels was seen in both the selected groups i.e endurance athletes and sedentary subjects after the exercise.

Lee et al. (2012) carried out a study on Korean population to examined the effect of 16 week Yoga practices on anthropometric parameters, adiponectin levels and metabolic syndrome factors in postmenopausal women with obesity. The results showed that after 16 weeks of Yoga practices there was significant reduction in BMI, % of body fat, weight, waist circumference, total cholesterol, low density lipoprotein, triglyceride and insulin resistance. Also, adiponectin and high density lipoprotein was found to be significantly increased. The authors concluded in their study that Yoga practice might be helpful in inhibtion of caridiovascular diseases in postmenopausal women with obesity.

Lee et al. (2014) examined the effect of 12 weeks Yoga on back pain, BDNF and serotonin levels in chronic low back pain premenopausal women. The result of the study revealed that in Yoga group back pain was significantly reduced whereas flexibility of back and BDNF levels was significantly improved along with maintenance of serotonin levels. In contrast, control group shows elevation in back pain and decline in BDNF and serotonin levels.

Lupine (1999) revealed in their study that decline in intellectual processes is associated with human aging. Moreover, some biological factors may be also related with cognitive aging like HPA, which control the system of stress hormones. They further explained that a brain structure involved in both human and animals, which is associated with learning and memory. They also know the impact of dementia and depression which increases glucocorticoid secretions in individuals.

Madanmohan et al. (2012) investigated the impact of 6 weeks (3 times per week) Yoga intervention on pre and post menopausal women with T2D by testing their biochemical profile and reaction time. The result of the study reported that after receiving Yoga training, auditory reaction time (ART) was improved for both the hands. However, statistically significant improvement was seen when ART was done with right hand. Furthermore, the improvements in glycemic profile (FBS and PPBS) and lipid profile (low density lipoprotein, total cholesterol, triglycerides, very low density lipoprotein and high density lipoprotein) were also observed after Yoga intervention.

Marek et al. (2011) in their study revealed that angiogenin concentration in vitreous and serum samples of the patients with T1Dplayed significant role in Diabetic retinopathy. Low vitreous concentration of angiogenin in Diabetic patients suggested that this component is not responsible for pathological neovascularization in Diabetic eye. More studies will make clear if angiogenin can be beneficial in

44

improving the insufficient angiogenesis in Diabetes and prevent retinal ischemia after retinopathy treatment with anti-VEGF agents.

Mcdermott et al. (2014) studied the efficacy of Yoga on people at high risk for Diabetes. The subjects were randomly divided into two groups i.e. Yoga and walking control group for 8 weeks. In Yoga group, after 8 weeks, the significant decrease was found on anthropometric variables i.e. weight, BMI, waist circumference in comparison to the walking control group. However, no significant differences were found among both the groups on the risk factors related with Diabetes viz; PPBS, FBS, insulin resistance and psychological well being. In addition, both the groups showed decline in total cholesterol, systolic blood pressure, diasystolic blood pressure, perceived stress, anxiety and depression. This study support the beneficial role of Yoga in controlling the anthropometric basis of risk factors associated with Diabetes.

Mullur and Ames (2016) have evaluated the impact of a 10 minute seating Yoga practices in the management of Diabetes. Totally 10 patients were recruited in this study with T2Dage ranges between 49-77 years. The Yogic intervention was given for 3 months and results shown improved health outcomes in Diabetes by routine Yogic practice combined with standard care.

Nagarathna et al. (2012) study focused on exploring the effect of two life style modification program (1) Yoga-based life style modification program (2) exercise-based life style modification program; on Diabetic Subjects (>28 Years) from Bengluru, India. The subjects were divided into Yoga-based life style modification program (include *asanas, pranayama*, meditation and lecture on Yoga) or exercise-based life style modification program (physical exercise and life style education) for nine months and assessment was done for medication scores, glycemic and lipid parameters. The result showed significant reduction in the intake of oral antidiabetic drugs, FBS and high density lipoprotein in Yoga group then exercise group. Moreover, both the intervention programs shows decline in glycated haemoglobin, very low density lipoprotein, blood glucose and total cholesterol.

Naveen et al. (2016) explored the possible correlation between BDNF and cortisol levels in depressive patients. The patients were divided into three groups i.e.

antidepressants group, Yoga therapy alone group and antidepressents + Yoga therapy group. The results show that in Yoga alone group negative correlation between BDNF and cortisol levels was seen in depressive patients. They further suggested in their study that Yoga therapy might be useful in improving neuroplasticity in patients with depression.

Neubaueret et al. (2012) in their study demonstrated that angiogenin levels are elevated in children and adolescent patients with T1D. The outcome of the study proved that Serum angiogenin level was lower in patients with T1D. In patients with clear Diabetic nephropathy, the angiogenin level was higher when compared to patients without nephropathy. They also concluded in their study that the presence of Diabetic microangiopathy, angiogenin level in middle-aged T1D patients is lower than in controls. The presence of overt nephropathy and smoking habit in middle-aged patients with T1D are associated with higher angiogenin level.

Nidhi et al.(2012) in their study revealed that Yoga was observed to be more valuable than physical activities in enhancing insulin, lipid, and glucose in adolescent girls with Poly Cystic Ovary Syndrome (PCOS). Results showed the changes in fasting insulin, FBS and insulin resistance were significantly different in the 2 groups. Moreover, the changes in blood lipid values were also significantly different (P<0.05) except for high-density lipoprotein cholesterol. However, no significant changes were found in BMI, waist and hip circumferences.

Nurnazahiah et al. (2016) studied the levels of adiponectin and leptin can be controlled by routine physical activity. Studies have revealed that physical activity are beneficial by controlling metabolic pathways and maintain the homeostasis by regulating the levels of adiponectin and leptin in in a wide range of adult groups.

Olaiya et al. (2019) carried out a study to know the impact of birthweight on early development (age <40 years) of T2D. The longitudinal study (1965-2007) was done on American Indians, and found that both the birth weight categories i.e. low and high were related with elevated risk of T2D in adolescents. They further added in their study that low birth weight category also related with increased possible risk for T2D at young adulthood.

Pascoe et al. (2017) reviewed that Yogic practices were correlated with decreased levels of systolic blood pressure, FBS, low density lipoprotein, resting heart rate, and cortisol levels (evening & waking in morning both) in comparison to the active control group. Moreover, Yoga practices were found to be associated with better functioning of HPA-axis and sympathetic nervous system.

Ramachandran et al. (2001) in their study evaluated the occurrence of Diabetes and IGT in six cities, representing every part of India. The assessments for oral glucose tolerance test OGTT was done on 11216 participants (age≥20 years). The authors found that 12.1% and 14.1% of the population was affected with Diabetes and impaired glucose tolerance respectively. Furthermore, Diabetes was positively correlated with growing age, WHR, BMI, genetic history of Diabetes and an inactive lifestyle whereas IGT was positively correlated with parental history of Diabetes, BMI and growing age. They also highlight in their study that higher occurrence of Diabetes was found in urban areas. In addition, huge number of people was on the verge of conversion from IGT to Diabetes.

Rani et al. (2011) focused on the evaluation of the impact of Yoga *Nidra* on psychological issues in females with menstrual disorders. One hundred fifty females with menstrual issues were randomly bifurcated in to two groups of experimental (N=75) and control (N=75) respectively. The data was collected pre and post six month yogic intervention. The results of the study revealed that anxiety and depression decreased significantly in the experimental (Yoga) group. Moreover, general health and positive wellbeing enhanced significantly in the Yoga group in comparison with the control group.

Rani et al. (2011) study focused on the treatment of patients with menstrual abnormalities by Yoga therapy. One hundred fifty females, with menstrual issues, were randomly bifurcated into two groups in various groups of experimental (N=75) and controls (N=75) respectively. The result showed that after the 6 months of Yoga therapy, there was significant improvement in pain symptoms (gastrointestinal symptoms, urogenital symptoms and cardiovascular symptoms) in comparison with control group. The outcomes of the study revealed that the side effects in patients with menstrual issue can be diminished by applying a Yogic program.

Rani et al. (2012) study focuses on to assessment of the impact of Yoga *Nidra* on anxiety and depressive manifestations in patients with menstrual issue. In this study subject was divided into two groups, one experimental group and another control group. The result of the study revealed that there was noteworthy decrease in scores in Hamilton anxiety scale (HAM-A) and Hamilton rating scale for depression (HAM-D) in subjects with anxiety and depression symptoms after following Yoga intervention for six months in experimental group in comparison to control group.

Ravikumar et al. (2011) revealed that HbA1c enhances with age. Their community based cross sectional study from Chandigarh above 20 years of age and showed the significant positive correlation between age of the subjects and HbA1c. The expansion in HbA1c with each growing year was 0.01% over the age of 20 years.

Reynolds et al. (2010) study was designed to assess the coginitve ability and estimate the lifetime changes associated with the fasting cortisol level in old age (65-70 years) individuals with T2D. The result of the study showed that higher fasting cortisol was related with noteworthy cognitive decline. In trial of working memory, handling speed, autonomous of mood, education, metabolic factors and cardiovascular diseases. They concluded in their study that higher cortisol levels in older individuals with T2Dwas associated with age-related cognitive changes. Moreover, they also suggested that by bringing down cortisol activity might be valuable in enhancing the cognitive decline in people with T2D.

Richardson et al. (1999) has revealed that VEGF which is involved in extracellular remodelling and angiogenesis, can be stimulated with the effect of exercise presumably due to intermittent hypoxia after exercise.

Richmond and Rogol (2016) study reveals the effect of exercise on neuroendocrine system in developing child. This study evaluated the changes during aerobic exercise in secretion of cortisol. Physical activity play vital role in strength of skeletal system before adolescence.

Saatcioglu (2012) explored how Integrative Medicine (IM) approaches have increased noteworthy enthusiasm for some years in order to answer the social challenges we confront today. Yogic psychological behavioural practices are among the most generally utilized IM approaches and incorporate different practices. For example, *Yogaasanas*, meditation, breathing activities, suggest that that these Yogic practices have huge constructive outcomes on the mind–body framework and in this manner can expand health and modulate diseases. This review concluded that Yogic practices have a measurable impact at the molecular level.

48

Satish and Lakshmi (2016) carried out a study on type 2 Diabetic patients to check the efficacy of 3 months Yoga in maintaining glycemic and psychological parameters. The assessment was done at 2 time points: pre and post test (3 months, 12 supervised sessions) of Yogic Practices. The result of the study revealed that significant decline was seen on FBS, symptoms and intensity of depression whereas significant improvement was observed on concentration, attention and QoL. However, no significant changes were seen in the variables of PPBS and glycated haemoglobin.

Schmalzl et al. (2018) investigated the impact of movement-focused practice and a breath-focused practice on sustained attention, cortisol levels and perceived stress among University students. The result of the study reported that perceived stress and cortisol levels got significantly declined in both the intervention groups whereas sustained attention was increased in breath focused group only. Moreover, negative correlation was found between sustained attention and perceived stress.

Selvam etal. (2017) carried out a training program on teachers and school children to impart health education on non-communicable diseases particularly Diabetes. A total of 1017 teachers from Tamilnadu, India were recruited for the study. Training included healthy lifestyle practices, prevention and management of Diabetes. It was found that 93.7% of the teachers responded positively and showed changes in knowledge and attitude. 60.4% students avoided unhealthy diets (Junk foods). This short term training programme resulted into significant awareness amongst both teachers and students.

Shiju et al. (2019) carried out a study on 5 day *Sudarshan Kriya* Yoga (SKY) on QoL, anxiety and depression in T2D. Moreover, they also assessed the 15 week impact of SKY on glycemic parameters in the same group. SKY was found to be effective in managing neuropsychological problems like depression, insomania and anxiety along with QoL. However, no significant changes were seen on glycemic parameters (HbA1c).

Singh et al. (2007) evaluated the predominance and dispersion of the metabolic syndrome (MS) in adolescents going to school in the city of Chandigarh. In a community based cross sectional survey, a total of 1083 adolescents age ranged from 12–17 years were taken for the survey. The result of the survey revealed the overall

4.2 % prevalence of metabolic syndrome in adolescents. Furthermore, when the fasting plasma glucose cut-off was brought down to 5.5 mmol/l the prevalence of metabolic syndrome increase upto 5.8%. No gender difference was found in the dispersion study and study represents a severe risk to the present and future health of these youngsters.

Singh et al. (2019) aimed to understand the risk of T2Damong 290 young medical students. Indian Diabetes risk score was used to detect the risk status for Diabetes in medical students. About 77%, 22%, and 1% students were found to be low risk, moderate risk and high risk respectively. The significant correlation was seen among parental history of Diabetes, physical inactivity and BMI in males when associated with moderate to high risk for Diabetes.

Singh et al. (2019) investigated the impact of 3 months Diabetic Yoga Protocol (DYP) on biochemical, radiological and stress profile of pre-diabetic women. The result of the study revealed that HbA1c, glucose values and stress levels were significantly decreased after 3 month DYP practice. Although, no increase in fatty liver was seen among pre-diabetic women after DYP practice. The authors concluded in there study that DYP may play a promising role in inhibiting pre-diabetes to Diabetes conversion.

Strachan et al. (2011) revealed in their study that those people, who suffered from T2D, may have increased risk of developing dementia. In their study, they revealed the multifactorial probability in individuals with T2D on the etiology of dementia and cognitive impairment. The data in this study recommends that the brain of old age individuals with T2D may be defenceless against the impacts of intermittent and extreme hypoglycaemia. Another cognitive function involves rheological factors, inflammatory mediators and dysregulation of HPA-axis. The study also concluded that cognitive function ought to now be incorporated as a standard end point in randomized trials of remedial intercessions in individuals with T2D.

Sullivanet al. (2019) investigated the effects of two interventions i.e. power Yoga and stretch Yoga on cortisol levels in college women and found that cortisol levels was significantly reduced after performing both types of Yoga. The authors concluded in their study that Yoga is a promising way for stress reduction and improved well being.

Supriya et al. (2018) evaluated the impact of Yoga practices (3 Yoga sessions per week for 1 Year) on individuals with metabolic syndrome (high to normal blood pressure). Molecular analysis included leptin, chemerin (proinflammatory adipokines), adiponectin levels (anti-inflammatory adipokine). The assessments were taken at pre and post test (1 year) in experimental (Yoga group) and control group. The result of the study reported that proinflammatory adipokines were decreased significantly whereas anti-inflammatory adipokine elevated significantly. Hence, Yoga was found to be a useful therapy for managing metabolic syndrome via adipokine modulation.

Telles et al. (2014) studied the comparative effect of Yoga or walking (1.5 hour per day for 15 days) in overweight and obese individuals on selected variables. The result of the study revealed that in both the groups, a significant decline in total cholesterol, waist circumference, hip circumference and BMI was seen. However, Yoga practice group showed decline in leptin and low density lipoprotein whereas walking group showed decline in adiponectin and triglycerides levels. Hence, both Yoga and walking was found to be effective in overweight and obese individuals as depicted by lipid and anthropometric data analysis.

Thind et al. (2017) carried out a meta analysis (n= 23 studies) investigated the impact of Yoga practices on glycemic parameters in T2D young adults. The improvement in glycemic parameters like HbA1c, PPBS, FBS was seen after Yoga practices in comparison to the control group. Moreover, the positive effect of Yoga was also seen on BMI, WHR, cortisol levels, lipid parameters and blood pressure in comparison to the control group. Hence, Yoga practice is helpful in controlling glycemic parameters and other comorbidities related with T2D.

Tolahunase et al. (2017) evaluated the effect of 12 week Yoga and meditation based lifestyle intervention (YMLI) on cellular aging on healthy individuals. After 12 weeks of YMLI practices, it was found that metabotropic and cardinal biomarkers were significantly improved. Moreover, the mean values were significantly decreased for 8-Oxo-2'-deoxyguanosine (8-OH2dG), reactive oxygen species(ROS), cortisol,

Interleukin 6 (IL-6), telomerase activity, β-endorphin, BDNF, and sirtuin-1. Hence, YMLI practice played a major role in inhibition of cellular aging.

Vaibhavi et al. (2013) conducted a pilot study to understand the effect of 6 weeks residential program and 12 week home program of *Panchkarma* + Yoga intervention in T2D patients (N=12, 40-70 years) on glycemic and lipid parameters. The result of the study revealed that after 6 weeks PPBS, FBS, total cholesterol, triglycerides and HbA1c decreased significantly. Further, after 12 weeks score of Oral Hypoglycemic drugs and HbA1c declined significantly. The study also proved the efficacy of Ayurveda panchakarma + Yoga in improving glycemic and lipid profile.

Venugopal et al. (2017) investigated the impact of short term (10-days) Yoga practice on Diabetic and pre-diabetic subjects with respect to their FBS. A total of 1292 subjects from different states (Karnataka, Maharashtra, Gujarat, Rajasthan, and Tamilnadu) of India participated in the study. The assessment for Fasting Plasma Glucose (FPG) was taken at pre test and post time. The study reported the significant reduction in FPG in Diabetic and pre-diabetic subjects. Hence, Yogic interventions were found to be effective in reducing the FBG values in both Diabetic and pre-diabetic subjects.

Wabsitch et al. (1996) examined the regulation of leptin expression in cultured human adipocytes. The result of the study revealed that in completed separated human fat cells, insulin incited a measurement subordinate ascent in leptin protein. Cortisol at a close physiological convergence of 10–8 mol/l was found to potentiate this insulin impact by three times. Expulsion of insulin and cortisol, separately, was trailed by a quick reduction in leptin expression, which was reversible after readdition of the hormones. These outcomes plainly show that both insulin and cortisol are strong and perhaps physiological controllers of leptin expression in human fat tissue.

Yadavet al. (2018) explored the comparative effect of 12 week Yoga based life intervention group with dietary intervention group on leptin, interleukin-6, 8-hydroxy-2'-deoxyguanosine, adiponectin and superoxide dismutase in Indian adults within the age group of 20-45 years with metabolic syndrome. The result of the study highlights that significant decline was found on the levels of leptin, 8-OH2dG, IL-6 whereas adiponectin and superoxide dismutase showed the elevated levels in Yoga based life

52

intervention group. Whereas, in dietary intervention group, no significant changes were observed which further emphasize the fact that Yoga based lifestyle intervention had better potential to improve oxidative stress in comparison to the dietary alone intervention group.

Yang et al. (2011) carried out a pilot study to examine the comparative effect of two intervention programs; (1) Yoga intervention group who received the intervention for 2 times per week and (2) educational group received educational materials on general health for every 2 weeks. Both the intervention programs were given for 3 months to the adults (45-65 years) with T2D risk. The study subjects (N=23) were divided into Yoga intervention group (N=12) and educational group (N=11). Between both the groups, the Yoga group showed improvement in blood pressure, weight, triglycerides and insulin levels. Hence, Yoga has a potential for reducing the cardio metabolic risk factors among adults.

CHAPTER – III
METHODS AND PROCEDURES

In this chapter, the design of the present study, selection of subjects, selection of variables, administration of tests, training regime, procedure of data collection and statistical procedure required for analysis of data was discussed.

3.1   DESIGN OF THE STUDY

The present research was conducted by using experimental research design. In the present study, 211 pre-diabetic/high risk women (≥60) were selected on the basis of IDRS. The selected participants were divided into control (N=81) and Diabetic Yoga Protocol (DYP) group (N=130). The selected volunteers in DYP group performed DYP approved by Ministry of AYUSH for three months (six times in a week) after signing written informed consent. Patient information sheet (PIS) was also provided to the participants. The control group continued to follow their daily regimen. The pre and post-test data was collected for the selected biochemical, molecular, neuropsychological and anthropometric parameters at baseline (pre-test) and after 3 months (post-test) as shown in Figure 3.2. The present study was carried out after the ethical approval taken from Institutional Ethics Committee, Panjab University, Chandigarh (PUIEC) and Institutional Ethics Committee, Postgraduate Institute of Medical Education and Research (IEC PGIMER). The present study was carried out under the strict guidelines of the Ethics committee of both the respective institutions.

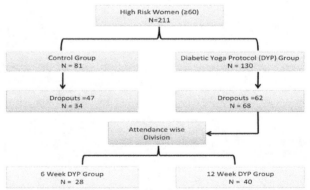

Figure 3.1: Flow chart showing detailed breakup of the samples. Dropouts are not considered for both control and DYP groups.

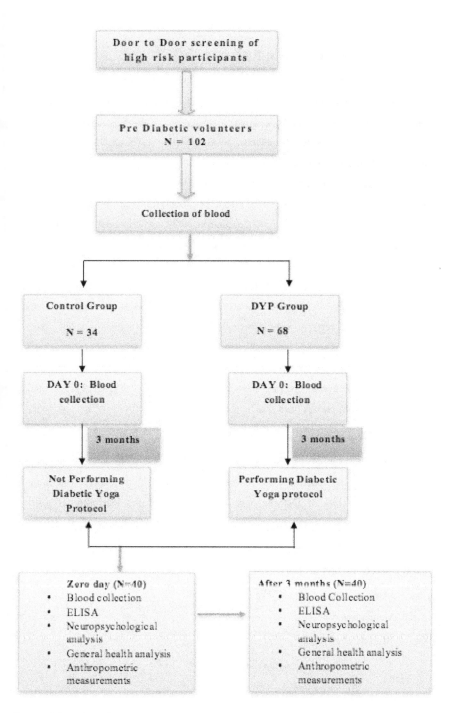

Figure 3.2: Flow chart showing the systematic procedure for data collection.

3.2   SELECTION OF THE SUBJECTS

The present study involves inclusion of volunteers based on IDRS. The subjects who scored ≥60 were included into the present study as they fall under the category of high risk (Mohan et al., 2005). A total of 211 high risk female volunteers of Chandigarh were selected as subjects from door to door screening. The total sample was divided into two groups i.e. one experimental (DYP) group (N=130) and one Control group (N=81). Further, after exclusion of the dropouts (Control Group- N= 47, Experimental (DYP) Group- N= 62) from the present study due to various reasons the total remaining sample was N=102 (Control- N=34, Experimental (DYP) group- N=68). The 68 female volunteers received DYP training for three months by experienced Yoga trainers, as experimental group. The experimental (DYP) group was further divided into 6 Week DYP group (N=28) and 12 Week DYP group (N=40) on the basis of attendance of the volunteers in the Yoga classes. The control group followed their daily regimen and did not receive any type of treatment or training. The subjects were assessed on selected anthropometric, molecular, biochemical and neuropsychological parameters before and after the Diabetic Yoga Protocol interventions .The age of the subjects will range from 20 to 70 years. The detailed break-up of the sample has been shown in Figure 3.1.

3.3   SELECTION OF THE VARIABLES:

On the basis of critical analysis of available literature as well as long discussion with the medical practitioners, scientists and Yoga experts and those working in the field of Diabetes and, consideration of the feasibility of tests, availability of the equipment and acceptability of the subjects following parameters were included for the present study.

3.3.1   Independent Variable:

Diabetic Yoga Protocol (DYP).

3.3.2   Dependent Variable:

(A)   Molecular markers

- Vascular Endothelial Growth Factor (VEGF)

- Brain-derived Neurotrophic Factor (BDNF)

- Angiogenin

56

(B)   Hormonal markers

- Leptin

- Cortisol

(C)   Biochemical variables

- Fasting Blood Glucose (FBG)

- HbA1c

(D)   Neuropsychological variables

- State Anxiety

- Perceived stress

- Sustained Attention

- General Health

(E)   Quality of Life (QoL)

(F)   Anthropometric variables

- Weight

- Waist Circumference

- Hip Circumference

- Body Mass Index (BMI)

- Waist Hip Ratio (WHR)

(F)   Risk analysis

- Indian Diabetes Risk Score (IDRS).

3.4   ETHICAL STATEMENT AND CONSENT:

The present study was conducted under the strict guidelines of institute ethical committee of Panjab University, Chandigarh and PGIMER, Chandigarh. The present study strictly followed all aspects of ethical guidelines approved by Institutional Ethical Committee, Panjab University, Chandigarh (No: PUIEC/2017/80/A-1/08/08, Dated: 06.12.2017) and PGIMER, Chandigarh (No: INT/IEC/2018/000184, Dated: 16.02.18). All the participants in experimental and control group were recruited by door to door screening (on the basis of IDRS) only after obtaining their written and /or audio-visual consent. The only invasive technique in the present study was used is blood withdrawal done at baseline and after 3 months (before and after). The information regarding the possible risk involved and its management in blood withdrawal procedure was provided to the participants through Patient Information Sheet (PIS).The possibility of complications is very less if proper procedure is followed. The experimental work was done under the GLP (Good Laboratory Practices) system maintained in the Neuroscience Research Lab, PGIMER, and Chandigarh. All the relevant research data and information related to the present study were kept in secured Laboratory environment. Moreover, the identity of the participants was also kept confidential. All the experiments conducted according to the Standard Operating Procedures (SOP) and further the all the acquired data thoroughly validated by QA (Quality Assurance) personnel.

3.5 ADMINISTRATION OF THE TEST

Subjects were selected for the present studies on the basis of IDRS score ($\geq$60). The pre and post test data was collected from the subjects with their consents. All the tests were administered by the researcher as per the requirements and procedure mentioned in the tools.

3.5.1 Diabetic Yoga Protocol (DYP)

The diabetic Yoga protocol approved by Ministry of AYUSH was used in the study, which is of 60 minutes in which 30 minutes were assigned to physical activity, another 30 minutes assign to pranayama and relaxation. The detailed description of the DYP is as under:

Table 3.1 Diabetic Yoga Protocol (DYP)

S. No	Name of Practice	Duration (min)
1	**Starting Prayer:** Asatoma Sat Gamaya	2
2	**Preparatory Sukshma Vyayamas and Shithililarna Practices** *1. Urdhavahastashvasan(Hand stretching breathing 3 rounds at 90°, 135° and 180° each)* *2. Kati-Shakti Vikasaka (3 rounds)* *a) Forward and Backward Bending b) Twisting* *3. Sarvangapushti (3 rounds clockwise, 3 rounds anticlockwise)*	6
3	**Surya Namaskara (SN)** 10 step fast *Surya Namaskara* 6 rounds 12 step slow *Surya Namaskara* 1 round **Modified version** Chair SN 7 rounds	9
4	**Asanas (1min per Asana)** *1 Standing Position (1min per Asana)* Trikonasana, Parvritta Trikonasana, Prasarita Padhastasana *2 Supine Position* Jatara Parivartanasana, Pawanmuktasana, Viparitakarani *3 Prone Position* Bhujangasana, Dharuasana followed by Pawanmuktasana *4 Sitting Position* Mandukasana, Vakrasana/ Ardhamatsayendrasana, Paschimatanasana, Ardha Ushtrasana At the end, relaxation with abdominal breathing in supine position (vishranti), 10-15 rounds (2 minutes)	15
5	**Kriya** a. *Agnisara*:1 minute b. *Kapalabhati(@60 breaths per minute for 1 minute followed by rest for 1 minute)*	3
6	**Pranayama** *Nadishuddhi(for 6 minutes, with antarkumbhak and jalandhar bandh for 2 seconds)* *Bhamari 3 minutes*	9
7	**Meditation** *(for Stress, for deep relaxation and silencing of mind)* **Cyclic Meditation**	15
8	**Resolve** *(I am Completely Healthy)*	1
9	**Closing Prayer:** Sarvebhavantu Sukhina............	1
	Total duration	60

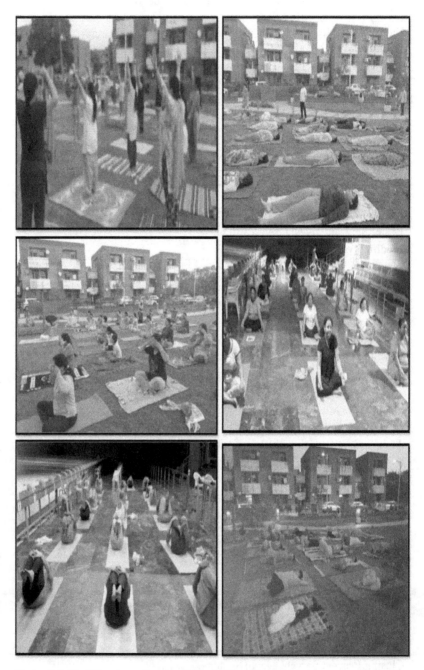

Figure 3.3: Participants performing Diabetic Yoga Protocol.

3.6   TESTS / TOOLS TO BE USED

In the current study, the data was collected with respect to different dependent variables like Biochemical, Anthropometric, Psychological and Molecular biomarkers. The tools / tests which were selected for measuring effect of Diabetic Yoga Protocol these variables are explained below.

3.6.1   Molecular and Hormonal Markers Assessment:

The estimation of protein level of selected molecular markers i.e. VEGF, BDNF, Angiogenin and hormonal markers i.e. Leptin and Cortisol were measured after collection of blood as follows:

Purpose: To estimate the protein level of the selected molecular and hormonal markers from blood serum.

a.   **Serum Separation**:

3.0 ml of blood was collected by a trained phlebotomist in a serum separator tube (SST) and was kept at room temperature (RT) for 30 minutes after collection of blood samples. After that blood samples were subjected to centrifugation for 30 mins at 2500 rpm for separation of serum from whole blood. Serum (upper separated layer) was collected in eppendorf tubes and stored at -80^0C within 1 hour of sample collection until assayed. Moreover, the whole procedure for blood sample collection and serum separation is shown in Figure 3.4.

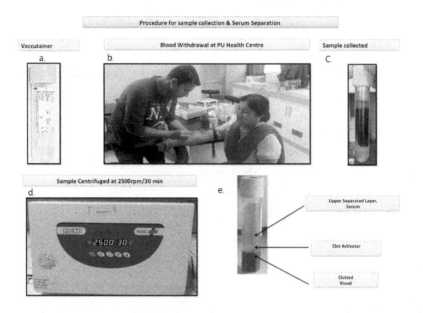

Figure 3.4 Procedure for sample collection and serum separation. **a.** Serum separator tube (Vacutainer) **b.** Blood withdrawal by the phlebotomist at PU health centre **c.** Blood sample collected in serum vacutainer **d.** Blood sample centrifuged in Remi centrifuge at 2500rpm for 30 minutes **e.** Serum separated.

Enzyme Linked Immuno-sorbent Assay (ELISA):

The protein levels of the serum samples were assessed by ELISA by using commercially available Elisa Kits (Qayee Bio, China). The procedure followed for the assessments of protein level in the serum was as per manufacturer's instructions. Before conducting ELISA experiment the samples were diluted, according to dilution factor. The prepared standards, diluted samples and HRP was added into ELISA plate and incubated for 1hour at 37^0C.After 1 hour the plate was washed with 1X wash buffer for atleast 5 times. After that available substrates were added and the plate was again incubated for 30 minutes at 37^0C. After incubation, stop solution was added and absorbance reading was taken at 450nm and the standard curve was made by using quadratic and linear model. The final values were normalized by total protein values in order to analyse and compare the protein levels in the samples. Moreover, Angiogenin, VEGF, BDNF and Leptin were estimated by sandwitch ELISA method and Cortisol by Competitive ELISA method. The detailed ELISA procedures shown in Figure 3.5

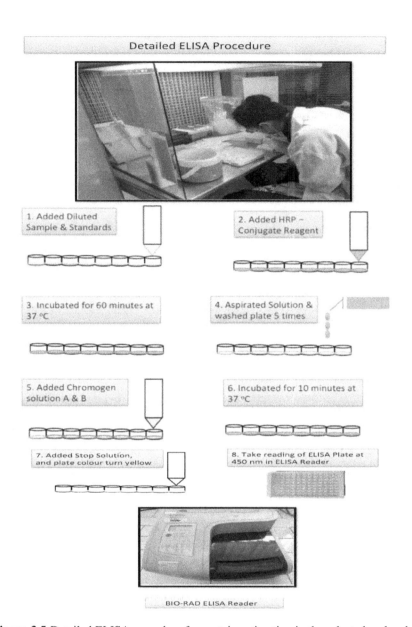

Figure 3.5: Detailed ELISA procedure for protein estimation in the selected molecular markers.**1.** Added 50 µl of standard & diluted samples in each well **2.** Added 50 µl of HRP conjugate reagent to each well. **3.** Incubated for 1 hour at 37^0C. **4.** Aspirated the solution and 5 times wash with washing buffer **5.** Firstly, add 50µl Chromogen A and 50µl Chromogen B solution to each well **6.** Incubated for 10 minutes for 37^0C. **7.** Added 50µl of stop solution to each well **8.** Taken reading of ELISA plate at 450 nm on ELISA reader. This is the illustration for the ELISA procedure for VEGF and BDNF according to QAYEE-BIO ELISA kit and procedure for other molecular markers are according to manufacturer instructions.

Estimation of Protein levels of the genes

The expression level of protein in selected genes was assessed in the pre-diabetic and control participants through serum by using commercially available ELISA kits for the selected genes. The absorbance reading for ELISA was taken at 450 nm. The protein values of the measured samples were neutralized by the values of estimated total protein.

C.   Total Protein Estimation

The total concentration of protein in the serum samples was estimated by using Bradford's reagent for normalization of selected candidate proteins, assessed by the ELISA. Samples were diluted with distilled water by a dilution factor of 400. For preparation of standards, Bovine serum albumin (BSA) was used. The concentration of standards was prepared within the range from 1000 to 15.62 ug/ml, which was further used for plotting of standard plot. The 10ul prepared standards and diluted samples were added into the respective wells in triplicates. The Bradford's reagent was diluted (1:5 times) by using distilled water and further 200ul of diluted Bradford's reagent was added into the wells. After 10-15 minutes of incubation at room temperature the absorbance reading was taken at 595 nm by using ELISA reader (Biorad). The standard curve was made by using linear fit models. The detailed total protein procedure shown in Figure 3.6

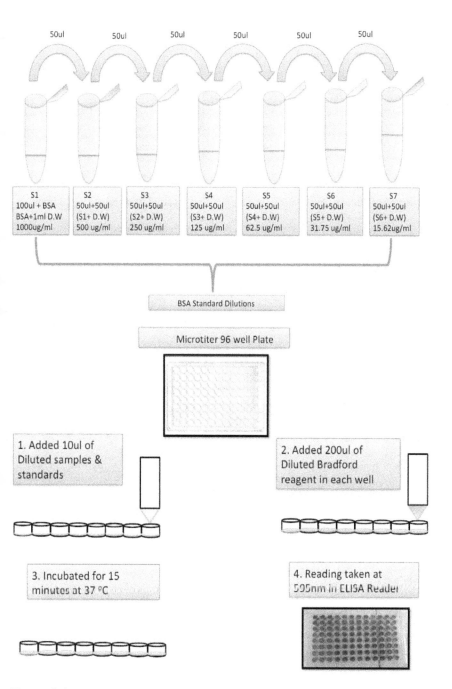

Figure 3.6: Showing the detailed procedure for total protein estimation from the samples.

3.6.2 Neuropsychological Assessments:

The selected psychological variables i.e. Perceived stress, Sustained attention, State anxiety was measured as follows:

Perceived Stress Scale (PSS): The perceived stress was measured in the participants by using Perceived Stress Scale (PSS) developed by Cohen et al. (1994). The PSS consisted of 10 item questionnaire at a 5 point likert scale. The questions asked in this scale are about the feeling and thoughts of the respondents regarding how stressful was their lives in the last month.

Purpose: To measure perceived stress of the participants.

Procedure: The subjects were asked to sit comfortably and then to rate the amount of stress they felt in the last month on the 5 point likert scale from never, almost never, sometimes, fairly often to very often. The respondents were asked to circle the response, which they felt most related to their feeling.

Scoring: The responses in the scale ranges from never (0) to very often (4). The scale consist of 6 negative items and 4 positive items and the reverse scoring was done for positive items. The final score was obtained by adding the scores of all positive and negative items. The range of scores for PSS is 0 to 40. Higher the scores show higher level of stress in the individuals as shown in Figure 3.7.

Validity: 0.52 to 0.76

Reliability: 0.84 to 0.86

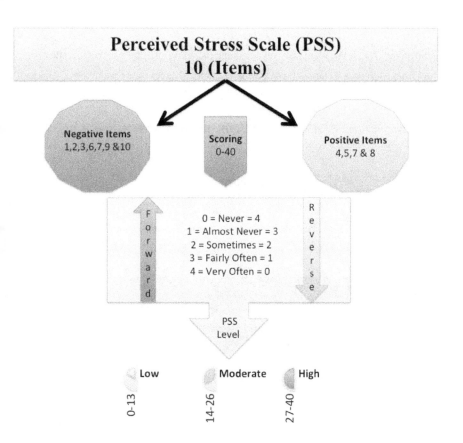

Figure 3.7: Detailed scoring procedure for measuring perceived stress by Perceived stress scale.

Six Letter Cancellation test (SLCT): Sustained attention was measured by using six letter cancellation test developed by Natu and Agarwal, (1997). SLCT is designed to focus upon performance of task with repetitive rapid response along with visual selection.

Purpose: To measure the selective and focused attention of the participants.

Procedure: Are searcher demonstrated (to the participants) the procedure for six-letter cancellation task. To avoid any ambiguity in the mind of the participants regarding the task, on the instruction of 'start', the participants needed to cancel the targeted six letters mentioned on the sheet (14 rows and 22 columns) as many as possible within the time frame of 90 seconds. Further, after the instruction of 'stop' the participant stopped the task. Moreover, the detailed procedure of SLCT is shown in the Figure 3.7.

Scoring: The final score was obtained on the basis of total number of attempts subtracted by total number of wrong attempts. Higher score shows the higher attention level of the participants. The scoring procedure also shown in Figure 3.8.

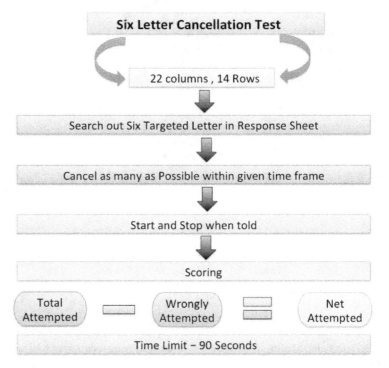

Figure 3.8: Detailed scoring procedure for measuring attention by Six Letter Cancellation test (SLCT).

Reliability: 0.78

Validity: 0.53

State and Trait Anxiety Test (STAI): State Anxiety was measured by using a sub-scale of state and trait anxiety inventory (STAI) constructed by **Spielberger** (1983, 2010). The Questionnaire is divided into two sub scales. The state Anxiety of the individual was measured by using a subscale (STAI Y-1). Questionnaire consisted of 20 questions to know the current anxiety related feelings of the participants. The scale is 4 point rating scale self report questionnaire.

Purpose: To measure the state anxiety (present feeling) of the individual.

Procedure: The subjects were asked to express their present feeling of anxiety among the four options (not at all, somewhat, moderately so & very much so) and tick the most relevant option describing their current feelings.

Scoring: This scale had 10 positive and 10 negative items. The joint score of positive and negative items shows the level of state anxiety in the respondents. The reverse scoring was done for negative items. The score is ranged from 20-80. The detailed procedures for scoring was also mentioned in Figure 3.9

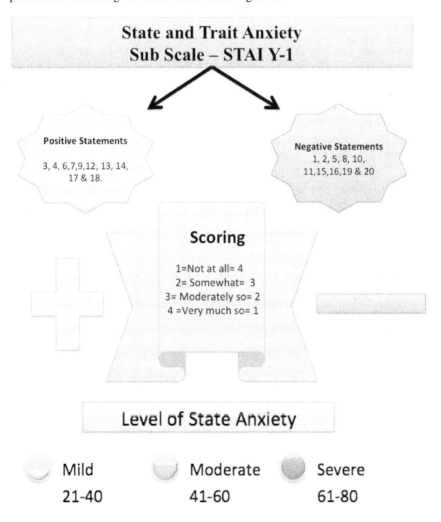

Figure 3.9: Detailed scoring procedure for measuring state anxiety by using a subscale of state and trait anxiety inventory (STAI-Y-1).

Reliability: 0.86-0.95

Validity: 0.73-0.85

3.6.3 General Well Being Assessment:

The selected general well being variables i.e. General Health and QoL were analysed as follows:

General Health: General health was analysed by General Health Questionnaire-12 (GHQ-12) developed by Goldberg et al. (1997). GHQ-12 is the 12 item self report questionnaire which asks questions about the problems (psychological) faced by the individuals presently or from some past weeks.

Purpose : To measure the general health level of the individual.

Procedure : The subjects were asked to tick among the four given options (More than usual, Same as usual, Less than usual & Very less than usual) which was most relevant to the respondents condition .

Scoring: The score is ranged from 0 to 36. The statement number 1,3,4,7,8,12 was scored like 0= More than usual,1=Same as usual,2=less than usual & 3=Very less than usual whereas statement number 2,5,6,9,10,11 was score reversely. The higher the score the worst is the individual's psychological health. The detailed procedure for scoring was mentioned in Figure 3.10.

Reliability: 0.87

Validity: -0.56

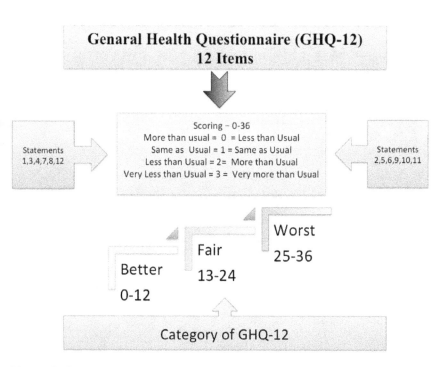

Figure 3.10: Detailed scoring procedure for measuring general health by General Health Questionnaire.

Quality of life (QoL): QoL was analysed by using WHOQOL (World Health Organisation Quality of life) scale (2004).The questionnaire consists of 26 questions on 5 point Likert scale and divided into four domains viz. Physical domain, Psychological domain, Social domain and Environmental domain.

Purpose: To measure the total QoL and it's associated domains.

Procedure: The subjects were asked to fill the questionnaire and out of 5 given options circle the most appropriate option that best describe their feelings or state.

Scoring : Firstly, the scoring for statement numbers 3, 4 and 26 was reversed and scoring of remaining statements was taken as such. Secondly, the domain (Physical, Psychological, Social & Environmental) wise scoring was done on the basis of equations shown in Figure 3.11. The obtained raw scores for each domain were further changed into transformed scores mentioned in the manual. The final score was obtained by adding the score of four mentioned domains, which further reflects the total Quality of Life of the participants. Higher scores denote higher QoL in the participants as shown in Figure 3.11.

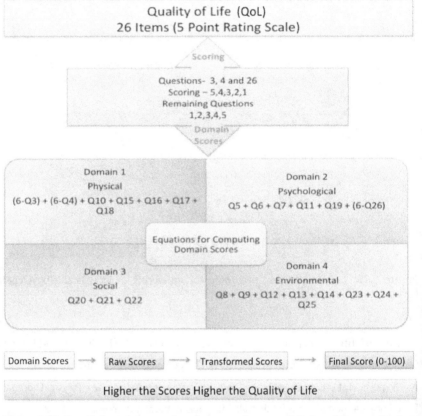

Figure 3.11: Detailed scoring procedure for measuring overall QoL and its associated domains by WHOQOL scale.

3.6.4 Risk Assessment: Indian Diabetes Risk Score (IDRS): IDRS is a simple, convenient, user friendly and economic method for screening of undiagnosed diabetic population or individuals who are at risk for onset of Diabetes develops by Mohan et al.(2005). IDRS screening was based on the four factors (age, waist circumference, physical activity and Diabetic family history) that contribute a major portion for prediction of risk factors associated with metabolic syndrome.

Purpose: To check the level of risk for development of Diabetes among the community.

Procedure: Firstly, the details about the age, Parental history of Diabetes and Level of physical activity was taken from the participants. After that Waist Circumference was measured with the help of measuring tape. The waist measurement was taken from above the naval region without compressing of soft tissue.

Scoring: The Indian Diabetes Risk Score (IDRS) was determined by adding the scores for each risk factor (high risk ≥60, moderate risk 30–50, low risk < 30). The scoring procedure was mentioned in Figure 3.12.

Sensitivity – 62.2 %

Specificity - 73.7%

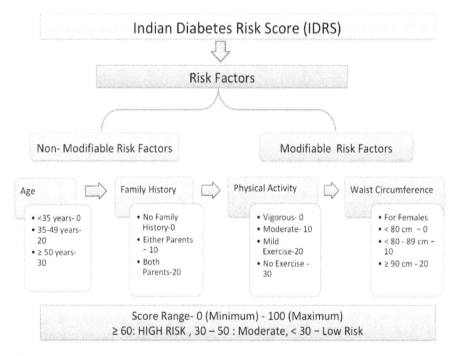

Figure 3.12: Detailed scoring procedure for measuring Diabetes risk status of the individual by using Indian Diabetes Risk Score (IDRS).

3.6.5 Anthropometric Assessment:

Height (H in cm):

The height of the participants was measured by using Stadiometer. The participants need to stand on the platform of the Stadiometer without shoes with weight equally distributed on both the legs along with legs joining their ankles. The sliding horizontal head piece was adjusted to rest on top of Head. The final reading of the height was taken where the sliding horizontal headpiece presses the head strongly.

a) **Weight (W in Kg):** The weight of the individuals was measured by using electronic weighing machine. The measurement was taken during minimal or light clothing, without shoes or removal of wallet or watch etc.

b) **Body mass Index (BMI):** The BMI is calculated by the following formula:

$$BMI= \text{Body weight (in Kg)/ Height}^{2} \text{ (in m}^{2})$$

c) **Waist Circumference (WC in cm):** The WC of the individuals taken from nearest 0.1 cm in a horizontal plane midway between the interior costal margin and the iliac crest. The measurement was taken with the help of measuring tape, which was fitted around the abdominal area without compressing soft tissue.

d) **Hip Circumference (HC in cm):** The HC was taken with the help of measuring tape and the measurement was taken around the maximum bulge from the buttocks.

e) **Waist Hip Ratio (WHR):** The WHR was calculated by the smaller circumference of the waist (above the belly) and dividing by the Hip circumference at the widest part of hip. The WHR was calculated by using the formula:

WHR = Waist divided by Hip (Waist / Hip).

3.6.6 Biochemical Assessments:

Biochemical variables i.e. FBS and HbA1c% was measured after blood collection by trained phlebotomist and done at the diagnostic laboratory using standard diagnostic procedures. The Fasting blood sugar (FBG) (Rxl-Max 500) was measured in early morning after 10-12 h of fasting. Level of HbA1c (Bio-Rad D-10) was also estimated.

3.7 COLLECTION OF DATA

For collection of data on various parameters (Molecular Markers: VEGF, BDNF, Anigogenin, Leptin and cortisol, Biochemical: FBG and HbA1c; Antropometric: Height, Weight, WC, HC, BMI and WHR; Risk: IDRS; Psychological

Assessment: State Anxiety, Perceived Stress, General Health, QoL, Sustained Attention) the high risk individuals on the basis of Indian Diabetes Risk score by door to door screening in the community were screened. The individuals with score of ≥ 60 were included in the study for three months after their written consent was obtained. Before the Pre-test, a meeting of all the subjects was held to explain them the purpose and objectives of the present study. The subjects were further asked for their solicited cooperation for the successful completion of the study. The participants were provided with Patient Information Sheet (PIS) in which details about the training regimen and testing procedures was mentioned. During the experimental period of three months, the subjects were not offered or advised any physical activities. The selected subjects underwent various molecular, biochemical, psychological and anthropometric assessments. The pre-tests and post-tests were taken after the period of 3 months.

3.8   STATISTICAL PROCEDURE

The data was analyzed by using SPSS Statistics, version 22.0 (IBM Corp., Armonk, New York, United States of America). The normality of the data was examined by using Kolmogorov's Simonorov test. The data was normally distributed. The paired t-test was applied to see the significant differences of means at pre test and post-test in pre-diabetic women in experimental and control group. The comparison of significance of differences for multiple markers in three tested groups i.e. control, 6 Week DYP and 12 Week DYP group was performed by One way ANOVA (Analysis of variance) followed by Tukey's post-hoc test when the null hypothesis was rejected. Further, Analysis of Covariance (ANCOVA) was carried out to test the significance of differences in the presence of covariates by treating post score as dependent variable, groups (Control/DYP and Control/6 weeks DYP/12 weeks DYP) as fixed factor and pre-scores and age as covariate. The level of statistical significance was set at ≤ 0.05.

CHAPTER - IV
ANALYSIS OF DATA, INTERPRETATION OF
RESULTS AND DISCUSSION

The present chapter is devoted to the presentation of results, their interpretation and discussion of findings in separate captions.

The present study was conducted 102 pre-diabetic women belonging to Chandigarh (U.T). The groups were divided into control group and DYP (Diabetic Yoga Protocol) group. The attendance wise results analysis of the participants was also done. The attendance wise results were prepared and the groups are divided into 6 weeks DYP group and 12 weeks DYP group and control group. The control group didn't undergo any training regime and followed their routine schedule. The purpose of the present study was to understand the effect of DYP on selected biochemical, anthropometric, neuropsychological parameters and molecular markers. The present study is experimental in nature, design to explore the effects of DYP on selected variables among the pre-diabetic population.

4.1   ANALYSIS OF DATA AND INTERPRETATION OF RESULTS

To measure the effects of experimental variable i.e. DYP on selected criterion measures: Molecular markers, Biochemical, Neuropsychological and Anthropometric parameters were taken for respective groups. The selected parameters were evaluated for significance by paired Student 't' test. The level of significance was set at ≤ 0.05.

76

Table 4.1: Pre-Post test mean comparison in control and DYP group on biochemical parameters i.e. Hba1c and FBG in mean, SD, and t- value with p- values.

Biochemical Parameters	Test Condition	Mean	SD	95% CI		t-value	p-value
				Lower	Upper		
HbA1c DYP Group	Pre-test	5.64	0.50	0.04	0.19	2.96	**0.004**
	Post-test	5.52	0.49				
FBG DYP Group	Pre-test	96.14	16.19	-9.58	0.37	-1.85	0.069
	Post-test	100.74	20.32				
HbA1c Control Group	Pre-test	5.87	0.62	0.02	0.29	2.37	**0.024**
	Post-test	5.72	0.58				
FBG Control Group	Pre-test	96.81	16.81	-5.60	5.48	-0.02	0.983
	Post-test	96.87	17.28				

Data is expressed in mean, SD and statistical significance (*p<0 .004**, p< 0.024**), HbA1c- Glycated Haemoglobin, FBG- Fasting Blood Glucose, SD= Standard Deviation, CI- Confidence Interval, DYP- Diabetic Yoga Protocol.

4.1.1 Comparison of HbA1c and Fasting Blood sugar in Control group and DYP group after a period of 3 months: Table 4.1 postulated that HbA1c was found to be significantly reduced in the Yoga group with (mean ± SD = 5.64 ±0.50 to 5.52 ±0.49), p=0.004 and in case of FBG (mean ± SD = 96.14 ± 16.19 to 100.74 ± 20.32) values were elevated though not significantly p=0.069 after 3 months of DYP practice. However also there was a significant reduction in HbA1c from mean ± SD = 5.87 ± 0.62 to 5.72 ± 0.58, p=0.024 in the Control group and in case of FBG levels (mean ± SD= 96.81 ±16.81 to 96.87 ±17.28) were found to be almost similar having no significant mean difference (0.983). The above stated result were also depicted through bar diagrams in Figure 4.1

Discussion of the results:

The result Presented in Table 4.1 & Figure 4.1 revealed that there was significant difference between the pre–test and post-test result of DYP Group in relation to HbA1c. However, in case of FBG no significant mean difference was found between pre and post-test results after 3 months of DYP Training. The significant difference in the mean values of HbA1c in DYP group (experimental group) indicates that DYP training of three month has positive impact in controlling the alarming signal for the progression of Diabetes, which can be measured from level of HbA1c (pre-diabetic=5.7-6.4). Moreover, Diabetic Yoga Protocol includes practices like *suryanamaskara,* which is helpful in activating insulin secretion through brain signaling (Kumari et al., 2012). Further, the practice of *asanas* rejuvenates cells of pancreas and increase the activity of insulin receptors in muscles that is further helpful in better glucose uptake in the muscles and body cells (Thangasami et al., 2015). In addition, *Kapalbhati* also improves the functioning of β-cells present in pancreas through abdominal pressure generated during forceful exhalation (Raveendran et al., 2018).

The result of the present study also supported by the study conducted by Rammoorthi et al. (2019) which stated that in pre-diabetes, Yoga practice, shows positive impact on glycemic and lipid parameters. They further supported the fact that Yoga practices are an integrative and alternative method for managing T2D.

However, in case of FBG shows in Table 4.1 & Figure 4.1 no significant mean difference was found between pre and post test results after 3 months training of DYP in DYP group. The present result may be due to the reliability and validity of FBG test as compared to HbA1c, which is more reliable and considered to be 'Gold Standard' for measuring glycemic index of the individual (Nagarathna et al., 2020).

Moreover, the normal range of FBG in relation to pre and post-test results indicate that the DYP group in reference to FBG already falls in the normal category. The little difference between pre and post-test results was obtained it may be due to sampling error or some other related factors.

Though, control group (Table 4.1 & Figure 4.1) also show significant decrease in the pre and post result in HbA1c level .The reason may be attributed to the fact that the individual from the control group after being aware of their pre-diabetic status might have changed their dietary and life style which is usually outside the control of the researcher.

Apart from significant difference the control group still falls under the category of Pre-diabetic stage. However, in case of FBG no significant mean difference was found between pre and post-test results. As per the pre and post results of the FBG of control group, it indicates that the control participants already fall under normal category.

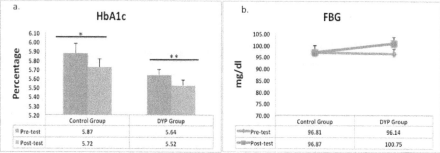

Figure 4.1 a) Mean changes in HbA1c levels for pre-test and post-test between control and DYP group *(p=0.004**, p= 0.024*)* **b)** Mean changes of FBG between pre and post for both the groups.

Table 4.2: Pre-Post test mean comparison within experimental (DYP) group on anthropometric parameters i.e. weight, BMI, WC, HC and WHR in mean, SD, mean difference and t- value with p- values in DYP group.

Anthropometric Parameters	Test Condition	Mean	SD	95% CI		t-value	p-value
				Lower	Upper		
Weight	Pre test	69.11	10.74	0.11	1.43	2.32	**0.024**
	Post test	68.35	10.99				
BMI	Pre test	28.64	4.31	0.05	0.59	2.40	**0.019**
	Post test	28.32	4.37				
WC	Pre test	93.46	9.06	0.60	3.24	2.90	**0.005**
	Post test	91.54	10.27				
HC	Pre test	104.09	9.77	0.33	3.09	2.47	**0.016**
	Post test	102.38	9.83				
WHR	Pre test	0.90	0.06	-0.01	0.02	0.63	0.530
	Post test	0.89	0.05				

Data expressed in mean, SD, and statistical significance *(p=0.005**, p=0.016*, p=0.019*, p=0.024*)* BMI- Body Mass Index, WC-Waist Circumference, HC- Hip Circumference, WHR- Waist Hip Ratio, SD= Standard Deviation, CI- Confidence Interval, DYP- Diabetic Yoga Protocol.

Table 4.3: Pre-Post test mean comparison within control group on anthropometric parameters i.e. weight, BMI, WC, HC and WHR in mean, SD, mean difference, and t-value with p- values in control group.

Anthropometric Parameters	Test Condition	Mean	SD	95% CI		t-value	p-value
				Lower	Upper		
Weight	Pre test	71.62	13.71	-0.01	1.53	2.01	0.053
	Post test	70.86	13.40				
BMI	Pre test	29.57	4.95	-0.02	0.61	1.91	0.065
	Post test	29.27	4.91				
WC	Pre test	96.39	12.96	-4.00	1.79	-0.78	0.443
	Post test	97.50	11.78				
HC	Pre test	103.79	12.51	-4.53	0.41	-1.70	0.099
	Post test	105.85	11.04				
WHR	Pre test	0.93	0.05	-0.02	0.03	0.61	0.548
	Post test	0.92	0.06				

Data expressed in mean, SD, and statistical significance; BMI- Body Mass Index, WC-Waist Circumference, HC- Hip Circumference, WHR- Waist Hip Ratio, SD= Standard Deviation, CI- Confidence Interval, DYP- Diabetic Yoga Protocol.

4.1.2 Comparison of the anthropometric parameters among the DYP group and control group after 3 months:

After 3 months of DYP practice (Table 4.2 & Figure 4.2) significant reduction in weight from 69.11±10.74 to 68.35±10.99 with p=0.024, and also BMI was found to be significantly decreased from 28.64 ± 4.31 to 28.32 ± 4.37 with p=0.019, along with WC with mean ± SD 93.46 ± 9.06 reduced to 91.54 ± 10.27, with p=0.005 and HC with mean± SD; 104.09± 9.77 reduced to 102.38±9.83, with p=0.016, also there was reduction in the WHR. However, the control group (Table 4.3 & Figure 4.2) has also shown reduction in weight (p= 0.053) and BMI (p=0.065) but not at significant rates.

And the WC (p=0.443) and HC (p=0.099) were increased in the control group post 3 months. And there was insignificant reduction in WHR (p=0.548) in the control group.

Discussion of the results:

The result present in Table 4.2 indicate that there were significant positive changes in DYP group for all the anthropometric parameters such as weight, BMI, WC and HC except Waist Hip Ratio. The result may be attributed to the fact that the DYP training programme consist of physical Yogic exercise, meditation and *pranayama* which put significantly reduce the weight of the practitioners resulting reduction in the BMI, WC and HC and also some positive changes in WHR.

The various studies have already supported the above said results on weight (Bernstein et al., 2014 and Kosuri and Sridhar , 2009), BMI (Zorofi et al., 2013), Waist Circumference (Ahn et al., 2006), Hip Circumferences (Kekan and Kashalikar, 2013) after Yogic practices. There are studies, which show no improvement in WHR (Hegde et al., 2013). In contrast there are some studies also available, which shows positive impact of Yoga on WHR (Ahn et al., 2006 and Keerthi et al., 2017).

During the Yogic classes the expenditure of energy increases along with mindfulness practices, which reduces the stress level among the practitioners resulting in less food intake, and the person feel more connected with their body which helps in maintenance of their body anthropometry (Bernstein et al., 2014).In control group, not involved in any physical activity, no significant improvements were seen on anthropometric parameters (Table 4.3 & Figure 4.2).

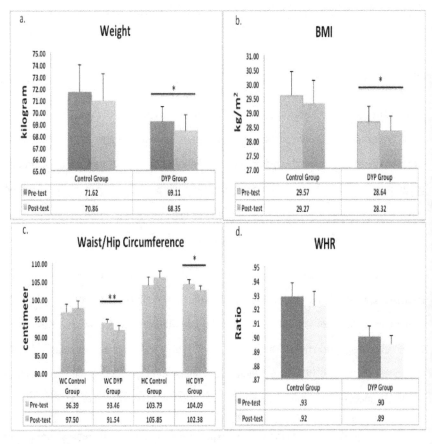

Figure 4.2 a) Mean changes in weight for pre-test and post-test for DYP group and control group *(p= 0.024*)* **b)** Mean changes in BMI for pre-test and post-test for DYP group *(p=0.019*)*. **c)**Mean changes in WC and HC for pre-test and post-test for DYP group and control group *(p=0 .005**, p=0.016*)*. **d)** Mean changes in WHR for pre-test and post-test for DYP and control group.

Table 4.4: Pre-Post mean comparison in DYP group on neuropsychological parameters i.e. sustained attention, general health, state anxiety and perceived stress in mean, SD and t- value with p- values at baseline (pre-test) and after 3 months.

Neuropsychological Parameters	Test Condition	Mean	SD	95% CI		t-value	p-value
				Lower	Upper		
Sustained Attention	Pre test	23.94	10.06	-8.43	-3.96	-5.57	< 0.001
	Post test	30.13	11.00				
General Health	Pre test	14.56	4.16	4.93	7.61	9.37	< 0.001
	Post test	8.29	3.37				
State Anxiety	Pre test	46.02	10.05	11.24	17.15	9.64	< 0.001
	Post test	31.83	8.18				
Perceived Stress	Pre test	19.65	6.47	4.62	8.14	7.24	< 0.001
	Post test	13.26	4.89				

Data expressed in Mean, SD, and statistical significance *p < 0.001****, SD= Standard Deviation, CI- Confidence Interval, DYP- Diabetic Yoga Protocol.

Table 4.5: Pre-Post mean comparison in control group at pre-test and post-test on Neuropsychological parameters i.e sustained attention, general health, state anxiety, perceived stress in mean, SD, and t- value with p- values at baseline (pre-test) and after 3 months.

Neuropsychological Parameters	Test Condition	Mean	SD	95% CI		t- value	p- value
				Lower	Upper		
Sustained Attention	Pre test	21.80	10.93	-6.76	1.96	-1.15	0.263
	Post test	24.20	14.24				
General Health	Pre test	13.65	2.80	-0.27	2.67	1.71	0.104
	Post test	12.45	2.44				
State Anxiety	Pre test	42.20	11.53	1.20	10.00	2.66	**0.015**
	Post test	36.60	10.18				
Perceived Stress	Pre test	18.91	5.52	-1.10	4.40	1.22	0.232
	Post test	17.26	7.25				

Data expressed in mean, SD, and statistical significance *(p=0.015*)* SD= Standard Deviation, CI- Confidence Interval.

4.1.3 Comparison of the re-test and post-test difference of Neuropsychological parameters in the DYP group and control group after 3 months:

Neuropsychological assessments (Table 4.4 & Figure 4.3) of the DYP participants showed significant improvement on all the selected neuropsychological parameters. General health shows significant reduction in the score with $p < 0.001$, with mean reduction from 14.56±4.16 to 8.29±3.37. State anxiety and perceived stress was also found to be significantly lowered found with mean score reduction from

46.02±10.05 to 31.83±8.18 with p < 0.001 for state anxiety and perceived stress score reduced from 19.65±6.47 to 13.26±4.89 at significant rates with p < 0.001. Interestingly, sustained attention score was significantly elevated after DYP with mean score elevation from 23.94±10.06 to 30.13±11.00 with p value of p < 0.001 in DYP group as shown in Figure 4.3 (b). The results on neuropsychological assessments has also been presented in Figure 4.3 (b)

Control group analysis of neuropsychological parameters (Table 4.5 & Figure 4.3) revealed significant reduction in state anxiety with mean reduction from 42.20±11.53 to 36.60±10.18 at p value 0.015. General health score was found to be reduced from 13.65 ±2.80 to 13.45±2.44 post 3 months with p=0.104. Sustained attention score was insignificantly elevated from 21.80±10.93 to 24.20±14.24. Perceived stress score were also found to be decline from mean 18.91±5.52 to 17.26±7.25 at insignificant rates.

Discussion of the results:

The Table 4.4 presented the pre and post results of experimental group trained on DYP in relation to neuropsychological changes which was observed on selected parameters that is sustained attention, general health, state anxiety and perceived stress through SLCT, GHQ, STAI and PSS test respectively. The results indicate positive significant changes in the neuropsychological behavior of experimental group who practiced three month DYP. The significant observed result may be attributed the fact that DYP consists of Yogic *asanas*, meditation and *pranayama* which directly work on the principle of developing harmonious coordination between sympathetic and parasympathetic nervous system which regulate the neuropsychological behavior of an individual.

Practice of *pranayama* help in controlling our breathing mechanism, which directly controls anxiety level and makes that individual more stable in perceiving any type of stress. Moreover, the practice of Yogic *asanas* improved general and psychological well being. (Kosuriet al., 2009; Sharma et al., 2008; Benavides and Caballero, 2009)

Our results are consistent with some another studies, which have shown improvements in sustained attention (Sarang and Telles, 2007), general health (Khemka et al., 2011) perceived stress (Hewett et al., 2018) and state anxiety (Satyapriya et al., 2013) after Yogic practices. Whereas the result presented in Table 4.5 indicate no significant mean difference between pre and post-test results on control group on selected neuropsychological (sustained attention, general health and perceived stress) parameters except in state anxiety (Table 4.5 & Figure 4.3). The significant mean difference found in state anxiety in control group may be due to the fact that as and when an individual became aware about their pre-diabetic status she became anxious but after the passage of time (three months) the post-test results, indicate that the subjects of control group accept this fact that they are in pre-diabetic condition. Moreover, the state anxiety associated with the current of the individual, which was depending on the different perceived and environmental situations.

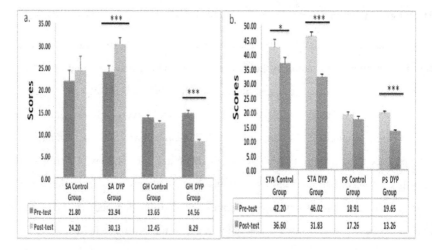

Figure 4.3 a) Mean changes in sustained attention and general health for pre-test and post-test for DYP group group *(p< 0.001 ***)* and control group;SA denotes Sustained attention; GH denotes General health **(b)** Mean changes in state anxiety and perceived stress for pre-test and post-test for DYP group group *(p< 0.001* and control group*(p<0 .015*)*;STA denotes State anxiety ; PS denotes Perceived stress

86

Table 4.6: Pre-post comparison in selected molecular markers like Angiogenin, VEGF and BDNF in mean, SD and t-values with p- values at baseline (pre-test) and after 3 months in DYP Group.

Molecular Markers	Test Condition	Mean	SD	95% CI		t-value	p-value
				Lower	Upper		
Angiogenin	Pre test	0.561	0.686	-0.361	-0.021	-2.24	**0.029**
	Post test	0.752	0.978				
VEGF	Pre test	0.0138	0.011	-0.004	-0.0003	-2.03	**0.046**
	Post test	0.0157	0.012				
BDNF	Pre test	56.43	93.96	-22.275	18.078	-0.21	0.836
	Post test	58.53	128.23				

Data expressed in Mean, SD, and statistical significance *(p<0.029*, p< 0.046*)* VEGF- Vascular Endothelial Growth; BDNF- Brain Derived Neurotropic Factor, SD= Standard Deviation, CI- Confidence Interval, DYP- Diabetic Yoga Protocol

Table 4.7: Pre-Post mean comparison in control group at pre-test and post-test on molecular markers i.e. angiogenin, VEGF and BDNF in mean, SD and t- value with p- values at baseline (pre-test) and after 3 months in Control group.

Molecular Markers	Test Condition	Mean	SD	95% CI		t-value	p-value
				Lower	Upper		
Angiogenin	Pre test	6.797	10.425	-0.833	3.406	1.24	0.226
	Post test	5.511	7.798				
VEGF	Pre test	0.0222	0.014	0.003	0.009	3.62	**0.001**
	Post test	0.0162	0.008				
BDNF	Pre test	34.97	36.85	-1.599	19.668	1.73	0.093
	Post test	25.94	36.79				

Data expressed in mean, SD, and statistical significance *(p=0.001**)* VEGF- Vascular Endothelial Growth; BDNF- Brain Derived Neurotropic Factor, SD= Standard Deviation, CI- Confidence Interval, DYP- Diabetic Yoga Protocol.

4.1.4 Comparison of the Pre-test and Post-test difference of Molecular markers in the DYP group and control group after 3 months:

Molecular markers of Angiogenesis and Neurogenesis were found to be significantly elevated after 3 month of DYP practice (Table 4.6 & Figure 4.4). Significant increase in angiogenesis markers that is angiogenin (0.561 ± 0.686 to 0.752 ± 0.978) and VEGF (0.0138 ± 0.011 to 0.0157 ± 0.012) was found with $p=0.029$ and $p=0.046$ respectively. Concentrations of BDNF (56.43 ± 93.96 to 58.53 ± 128.23) were also found to be elevated after DYP practice but not significant level ($p=0.836$).

However, in the control group (Table 4.7 & Figure 4.4) the Angiogenesis and Neurogenesis markers post 3 months were found to be reduced in VEGF (0.0222 ± 0.014 to 0.0162 ± 0.008) levels were significantly reduced ($p=0.001$) followed by reduced angiogenin (6.797 ± 10.425 to 5.511 ± 7.798) levels. And BDNF (34.97 ± 36.85 to 25.94 ± 36.79) levels were also insignificantly reduced after 3 months.

Discussion of the results:

The results postulated in Table 4.6 & Figure 4.4 shows the pre and post results of experimental group (DYP group) in relation to selected molecular markers, which are angiogenin, VEGF and BDNF shows changes in protein levels of selected molecular markers in DYP group after 3 months of DYP practice. The angiogenesis (angiogenin, VEGF) and neurogenesis (BDNF) markers showed increase in experimental group (DYP group) after 3 months of Yogic practice. The results presented in Table 4.6 indicate significant increase on angiogenesis markers in experimental group and also found some positive changes in neurogenesis markers (BDNF), which was measured through ELISA.

Tahergorabi et al. (2012) stated that angiogenesis is a process through which new blood vessels are formed through pre existing vessels which further facilitates oxygen and blood flow in the body. The result of increased angiogenesis markers may be attributed to DYP, consisting of various Yogic *asana,* specially of *Suryanamaskara,* may be responsible for increase in the blood flow and oxygen in the body may be taking place. The VEGF is the chief marker of angiogenesis, which promotes the process of angiogenesis in healthy and diseased conditions through signaling to VEGF receptor-2 (VEGFR-2) (Carmeliet and Jain, 2011).

Even the result of the present study is consistent with Vital et al. (2014) who explain the mechanism of elevated the blood on the exercised part due to physical and

Yogic exercises. A study done by Bloor et al. (2005) linked the increase in VEGF levels with rise and enlargement of artery and capillary respectively.

The systematic review done by Vital et al., 2014 on the effects of different exercise training programs on elder population found that, among the ten studies reviewed by the authors, four studies reported an elevated VEGF levels and six studies show no differences on the VEGF levels (Vital et al., 2014)

These studies supported the pro-angiogenic effect of exercise/Yoga and its impact on overall well being. The results of the present study open the new vista for exploring the role of Yoga on the phenotypic effects of various molecular markers.

BDNF is a potent factor in neuroplasticity, which has higher expression in brain, which is involved in survival and formation of neurons and linked with the cognitive functions of the individual. BDNF (neurogenesis) levels are also interlinked with the angiogenesis. The VEGF concentrations, which are activated by physical and meditative activity act as a mediator between angiogenesis and neurogenesis, (Cao et al., 2004; Cotman et al., 2007; Trejo et al., 2001 and Voss et al., 2013). VEGF is also essential for the stimulation of neurogenesis in the brain (Fabel et al., 2003).

In present study, the increase in mean levels of BDNF were seen in DYP group after 3 months of DYP practice but not at significant level. The positive impact of Yogic/physical exercises on BDNF levels might be due to its effectiveness in maintaining neuroendocrine balance by stimulating neurogenesis (Baptista, and Andrade, 2018). The Viver et al. (2012) in their study highlighted the fact that BDNF alterations after physical exercise influence the hippocampal plasticity. The meditative /Yogic practices enhance the hippocampal sizes/activity linked with BDNF concentrations (Holzel et al., 2008; Luders et al., 2009 and Gotink et al., 2016). A study done by Cahn et al., 2017 reported that Yoga and meditative practices are linked with the elevated levels of BDNF, which is further correlated with brain, and psychological wellness of the individual. The enhanced BDNF levels act as a facilitator between well being of brain and meditative practices (Cahn et al., 2017). There are some studies, which highlight the beneficial effects of Yoga on BDNF (Raju and Nagendra, 2017) and neuropsychological parameters (Hallappa et al., 2018).

Although the control group (Table 4.7 & Figure 4.4) demonstrated decrease in the mean levels of angiogenin, VEGF and BDNF levels but the significant decline in

VEGF levels was seen in control group. The decline in the levels of selected molecular markers in control group might be due to no treatment. There is also consistent with a study that the decrease in VEGF levels correlates with the pathological (pre-diabetes, obesity etc.) or diseased conditions of the individual (Prior et al., 2003). Moreover, decreased expression of VEGF in pancreatic beta cells can hamper the effectiveness of insulin and consequently lead to the pre-diabetic condition in adults.

The VEGF acts as a median between angiogenesis and neurogenesis and VEGF activate through physical activity (Cao et al., 2004; Cotman et al., 2007;Trejo et al., 2001 and Voss et al., 2013). However, in our study VEGF levels were reduced significantly in control group and VEGF didn't act as a mediator between angiogenesis and neurogenesis in control group which further results in the decline of mean levels of angiogenin and BDNF, which are the markers of angiogenesis, and neurogenesis, respectively.

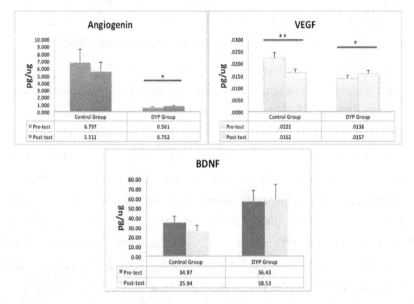

Figure 4.4 a) Mean changes in Angiogenin levels for pre-test and post-test for DYP group and control group *(p=0 .029*)*. **b)** Mean changes in VEGF levels for pre-test and post-test for DYP group and control group *(p=0 .046*, p=0.001**)*.**c)** Mean changes in BDNF levels for pre-test and post-test for DYP group and control group.

90

Table 4.8: Pre-Post test mean comparison in selected Hormonal markers i.e cortisol and leptin in mean, SD and t-value with p- values at baseline (pre-test) and after 3 months in DYP and control Group.

Hormonal Markers	Test Condition	Mean	SD	95% CI		t-value	p-value
				Lower	Upper		
Cortisol DYP Group	Pre test	0.0012	0.0011	-0.00091	-0.00007	-2.32	**0.024**
	Post test	0.0016	0.0014				
Leptin DYP Group	Pre test	0.00027	0.0003	-0.00006	0.00002	-0.90	0.374
	Post test	0.00029	0.0003				
Cortisol Control Group	Pre test	0.0017	0.0023	-0.00023	0.00103	1.30	0.202
	Post test	0.0013	0.0010				
Leptin Control Group	Pre test	0.00044	0.0003	-0.00011	0.00015	0.27	0.791
	Post test	0.00042	0.0004				

Data expressed in mean, SD, and statistical significance *(p<0.024*)* SD= Standard Deviation, CI- Confidence Interval, DYP- Diabetic Yoga Protocol

4.1.5 Comparison of the Pre-test and Post-test difference of Hormonal markers in the DYP group and control group after 3 months:

After 3 months of DYP practice (Table 4.8 & Figure 4.5) significant elevation in cortisol levels from mean ± SD = 0.0012± .00111) to mean ± SD = 0.0016±0.0014) with p−0.024 and also leptin levels were increased slightly from mean ± SD = 0.00027 ±0.0003 to mean ± SD = 0.00029±0.0003 but not at significant level with p=0.374. However, Cortisol levels show insignificant reduction from mean ± SD = 0.0017±0.0023 to mean ± SD = 0.0013±0.0010, p=0.202 in control group whereas leptin levels also shows non-significant reduction in control group from mean ± SD = 0.00044 ±0.0003 to mean ± SD =0.00042±0.0004, with p=0.202 (Table 4.8 & Figure 4.5).

Discussion of the results

The result of the present study presented in Table 4.8 & Figure 4.5 indicates significantly increased cortisol levels in experimental group (DYP group) after 3 months of DYP practices. The result of our study shows rise in cortisol levels in the subjects as sample was taken in the morning after 30-40 minutes of waking up. The cortisol levels are at its highest point after 30 minutes of waking up in early morning and also known as Cortisol awakening response (CAR) (Wust et al., 2000 and Cahn et al., 2017). Our study shows significant increase in cortisol awakening response, which is consistent with the results of the some other studies (Matousek et al., 2011 and Cahn et al., 2017). Cahn et al. (2017) associate cortisol-awakening response with increased alertness, and better quality of sleep, awakening in morning and stress reliever (Fries et al., 2009 and Clow et al., 2010).

As secretion of cortisol levels is based on diurnal cycle, which is highest in the morning and lowest in the midnight. Keeping in view this fact, we administered DYP training to experimental group in the morning, consisting of varied type of Yogic *asanas* mentioned in the Diabetic Yoga Protocol after performing warming up exercises and *suryanamskara*. All these Yogic practices stimulate the HPA axis pathway with the help of BDNF through hippocampal activation. A study shows the interconnectivity between BDNF and CAR and Yogic and meditative practice target CAR activity through stimulation of BDNF through hippocampal activation (Cahn et al., 2017).

In response to stress cortisol hormone was produced by Adrenal gland, which functioned as a constituent of hypothalamic-pituitary-adrenal (HPA) axis. The normal functioning of HPA axis levels is associated with elevated cortisol levels upon waking up, highest after 30-40 min of waking up and gradually declines during the course of the day and it is part of the circadian clock of the body. However, the abnormal functioning of HPA axis is linked with the psychological abnormalities (Curtis et al., 2011). In the pathogenesis, of Diabetes, cortisol levels play a major role and the activity of HPA is dramatically enhanced (Chiodini et al., 2007). Moreover, diurnal cortisol levels are correlated with the chances of developing Diabetes in near future (Hackett et.al. 2016).

Leptin plays major role in maintaining energy balance along with uptake of food and its metabolism in the body. It is further associated with fasting insulin levels. leptin levels were correlated with elevated body fat. There is a linkage shown between leptin and insulin resistance with pre-diabetes (Wang et al., 2010).

A study performed by Telles et al. (2009) on obese individuals reported that after Yoga Program, dietary modifications lead to decreased serum leptin (44.2%) levels (Telles et al., 2009). The meta analyses carried out by Yu et al., 2017 also shows beneficial effect of exercise on leptin and report that exercise significantly reduces serum leptin levels. In contrast, another study undertaken by Telles et al. (2014) did a comparative study on walking and Yoga for 15 days intervention and both the group showed decrease in BMI, waist circumference and hip circumference. The Yoga group showed increased serum leptin (p<0.01) and decreased LDL cholesterol (p<0.05). The walking group showed decreased serum adiponectin (p<0.05) and triglycerides (p<0.05). The increased leptin levels are associated with the leptin resistance in the obese people (Amitani et al., 2013).

Keeping in view of the literature available on the effect of Yogic exercise on leptin secretion more and more research work is required to be undertaken to validate the effect of exercise on leptin secretion. Though, control group shows no significant changes in cortisol and leptin levels, as they are not receiving any treatment (Table 4.8 & Figure 4.5)

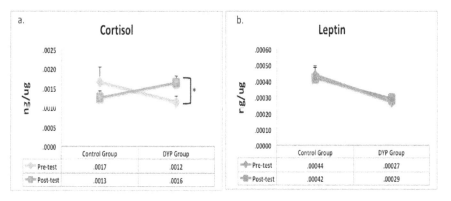

Figure 4.5 a) Mean changes in cortisol for pre-test (baseline) and post-test for DYP group and control group *(p<0 .024*)*. **b)** Mean changes in leptin for pre-test (baseline) and post-test for DYP group and control group.

Table 4.9: Pre-post test mean comparison in domains of Quality of Life (QoL) like Physical, Psychological, Social and Environmental domain and Overall QoL in mean, SD and t-value with p- values at baseline (pre-test) and after 3 months in DYP Group.

Domains of QoL	Test Condition	Mean	SD	95% CI		t-value	p-value
				Lower	Upper		
Physical Domain	Pre test	55.94	9.24	-8.66	-2.72	-3.85	< 0.001
	Post test	61.63	8.42				
Psychological Domain	Pre test	55.94	7.81	-9.68	-1.82	-2.94	0.005
	Post test	61.69	12.27				
Social Domain	Pre test	63.96	14.70	-16.98	-7.55	-5.22	< 0.001
	Post test	76.23	13.96				
Environmental Domain	Pre test	73.25	8.69	-13.97	-7.11	-6.17	< 0.001
	Post test	83.79	13.01				
QoL	Pre test	248.94	25.84	-45.09	-26.18	-7.57	< 0.001
	Post test	284.58	36.15				

Data expressed in mean, SD, and Statistical significance *(p< 0.001***, p=005),* SD= Standard Deviation, CI- Confidence Interval, QoL- Quality of Life DYP- Diabetic Yoga Protocol

4.1.6 Comparison of the Pre-test and Post-test difference of Overall QoL and domains of QoL in the DYP group and control group after 3 months:

The domains of QoL like physical (55.94±9.24 to 61.63±8.42, p< 0.001), psychological, (55.94±7.81 to 61.69±12.27, p=0.005) social (63.96±14.70 to 76.23±13.96,p< 0.001) and environmental domain (73.25±8.69 to 83.79±13.01, p< 0.001) with overall Quality of Life (QoL) (248.94±25.84 to 284.58±36.15,p< 0.001) shows significant increase after 3 months of DYP practice (Table 4.9 & Figure 4.6).

94

However, control group (Table 4.10 & Figure 4.7) also shows significant increase in overall QoL (248.75±32.62 to 260.35±35.93, p=0.030) and psychological domain (54.45±11.03 to 60.05±9.01,p=0.031) whereas non significant changes was seen in physical (57.90±7.09 to 57.60±7.04,p=0.814), social (65.60±16.50 to 67.50 ±13.83,p=0.516) and environmental domain (70.80±11.87 to 75.15±13.00,p=084).

Discussion of the results:

The result presented in Table 4.9 indicates significant improvement in the experimental group who had practiced DYP for three months. The present result may be attributed to the fact that significant improvement in the QoL and its domains is due to the effect of Yogic practices, which is a combination of *asanas, pranayama* and meditation practices an deals with synchronized collaboration of mind and body relationship.

The QoL incorporates the physical, psychological, social and environmental domain of the individual and Yoga found to be helpful in bringing positive changes in QoL and its domains. Yoga through *asanas, pranayama* and meditative practices bring positive effect on physical and psychological domain. The social and environmental domain also shows improvements which might be due to fact that during Yoga classes people enjoy the class and exchange their ideas and become more social and aware about their nearby environment. A study correlated the improvement in QoL with insulin signaling (Kleinridders et al., 2014) pathway in the hippocampal and prefrontal cortex region in the brain by stimulating serotonin neuronal pathway, which further bring changes in mood and behavior (Kleinridders et al., 2015). There are studies which shows significant improvement in Overall QoL after Yogic practices (Jyotsana et al., 2012; Shiju et al., 2019 and Keerthi et al., 2017)

However, control group also shows significant improvement in overall QoL and psychological domain but other domains like physical, social and environmental domain did not show significant improvements (Table 4.10 & Figure 4.7). The reason behind increase in QoL is might be the awareness about the pre-diabetic condition which insisting them to change their lifestyle.

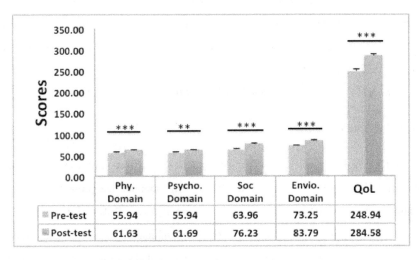

	Phy. Domain	Psycho. Domain	Soc Domain	Envio. Domain	QoL
Pre-test	55.94	55.94	63.96	73.25	248.94
Post-test	61.63	61.69	76.23	83.79	284.58

Figure 4.6 Mean changes in overall QoL and domains of QoL for pre-test and post-test for DYP. Phy -Physical domain, Psycho - Psychological domain, Socio- Social domain and Enviro- Environmental domain *(p< 0.001***, p= 0.005**).*

Table 4.10: Pre-Post test mean comparison in domains of QoL like physical, psychological, social and environmental domain and Overall QoL in mean, SD and Mean difference, t-value with p- values at baseline (pre-test) and after 3 months in control Group

Domains of QOL	Test Condition	Mean	SD	95% CI		t-value	p-value
				Lower	Upper		
Physical Domain	Pre test	57.90	7.09	-2.33	2.93	0.24	.814
	Post test	57.60	7.04				
Psychological Domain	Pre test	54.45	11.03	-10.62	-0.58	-2.33	**.031**
	Post test	60.05	9.01				
Social Domain	Pre test	65.60	16.50	-7.91	4.11	-0.66	.516
	Post test	67.50	13.83				
Environmental Domain	Pre test	70.80	11.87	-9.34	0.64	-1.82	.084
	Post test	75.15	13.00				
QoL	Pre test	248.75	32.62	-21.96	-1.24	-2.34	**.030**
	Post test	260.35	35.93				

Data expressed in mean, SD, and statistical significance *(p< 0.031*, p< .030*)* QoL- Quality of Life, SD= Standard Deviation, CI- Confidence Interval, DYP- Diabetic Yoga Protocol.

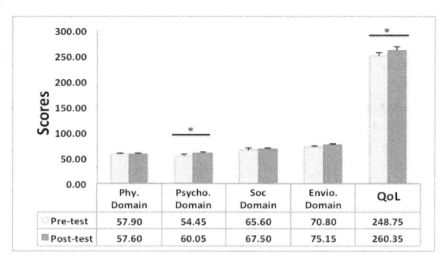

	Phy. Domain	Psycho. Domain	Soc Domain	Envio. Domain	QoL
Pre-test	57.90	54.45	65.60	70.80	248.75
Post-test	57.60	60.05	67.50	75.15	260.35

Figure 4.7 : Mean difference between overall QoL and domains of QoL for pre-test and post-test for control group. Phy -Physical domain, Psycho - Psychological domain, Socio- Social domain and Enviro- Environmental domain *(p< 0.31*, p< .030*)*

Table 4.11: Pre-Post test mean comparison in selected biochemical parameters like HbA1c and FBG in mean, SD and t value with p values in 6 weeks DYP Group and 12 weeks DYP Group.

Biochemical Parameters	Test Condition	Mean	SD	95% CI		t-value	p-value
				Lower	Upper		
HbA1c 6W DYP	Pre test	5.60	0.39	0.02	0.24	2.43	**0.022**
	Post test	5.47	0.39				
FBG 6W DYP	Pre test	90.55	11.86	-15.69	-0.49	-2.19	**0.038**
	Post test	98.64	22.61				
HbA1c 12W DYP	Pre test	5.67	0.57	-0.01	0.21	1.87	.070
	Post test	5.57	0.55				
FBG 12W DYP	Pre test	100.34	17.83	-8.77	4.79	-0.60	0.554
	Post test	102.33	18.58				

Data expressed in mean, SD, and statistical significance *(p=0.022*, p=0.038*)* HbA1c- Glycated Haemoglobin, FBG-Fasting Blood Glucose, SD=Standard Deviation, CI- Confidence Interval, DYP- Diabetic Yoga Protocol, 6W- 6 weeks, 12W- 12 weeks

4.1.7 Comparison of the Pre-test and Post-test difference of Biochemical Parameters in the 6 weeks DYP group and 12 weeks DYP group after 3 months:
Table 4.11 & Figure 4.8indicates the pre-post values for HbA1c and FBG after performing Yoga for 6 weeks and 12 weeks. The HbA1c (mean ± SD = 5.60 ± 0.39 to 5.47 ± 0.39, p- 0.022) decreased significantly and FBG (mean ± SD = 90.55 ± 11.86 to 98.64 ± 22.61, p- 0.038) increased significantly after performing Yoga for 6 weeks, whereas no significant difference was found between both the parameters after performing Yoga for 12 weeks, HbA1c (mean ± SD = 5.67 ± 0.57 to 5.57 ± 0.55,p- 0.070), FBG (mean ± SD = 100.34 ± 17.83 to 102.33± 18.58, p- 0.554) (Table 4.11 & Figure 4.8).

Discussion of the results:

The result of the present study revealed that 6 weeks DYP group shows significant differences on HbA1c and FBG in comparison with pre-test and post-test. In 6 weeks DYP group, HbA1c (p=0.022) shows significant improvement but FBG (p=0.38) demonstrates significant rise between pre-test and post-test. However, FBG mean value was within the normal range according to ADA guidelines. Surprisingly, the 12W DYP group shows no significant changes in HbA1c and FBG. The DYP group helps in maintaining the glycemic control in the participants. The HbA1c is considered as the most reliable for glycemic control, which shows the maintenance of normal category HbA1c in both the DYP groups. The comprehensive discussion of the same section has been also mentioned on section 4.1.1.

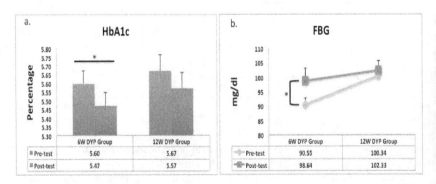

Figure 4.8 : a) Mean changes inHbA1c levels for pre-test and post-test for 6 weeks and 12 weeks DYP group *(p<0.022)*. **b)** Mean changes in FBG between pre and post test for 6 weeks and 12 weeks DYP group *(p<0 .038*)*

Table 4.12: Pre-Post test mean comparison in selected anthropometric parameters like weight, BMI, WC, HC and WHR in mean, SD and t-value with p- values at Pre-test and Post-test in 6 weeks DYP group.

Anthropometric Parameters	Test Condition	Mean	SD	95% CI		t-value	p-value
				Lower	Upper		
Weight	Pre test	70.25	11.93	-1.44	1.05	-0.32	.749
	Post test	70.44	12.27				
BMI	Pre test	29.10	4.88	-0.57	0.43	-0.29	0.771
	Post test	29.17	4.94				
WC	Pre test	93.89	10.11	-0.11	4.43	1.95	0.061
	Post test	91.73	11.80				
HC	Pre test	104.43	11.54	-1.27	3.19	0.89	0.383
	Post test	103.46	11.36				
WHR	Pre test	0.90	0.07	-0.01	0.04	1.10	0.280
	Post test	0.89	0.06				

Data expressed in mean, SD, and statistical significance BMI- Body Mass Index, WC- Waist Circumference, HC- Hip Circumference, WHR- Waist Hip Ratio, SD= Standard Deviation, Diff-Difference, CI- Confidence Interval, DYP- Diabetic Yoga Protocol, 6W- 6 weeks.

4.1.8 Comparison of the Pre-test and Post-test difference Anthropometric parameters in the 6 weeks DYP group and 12 weeks DYP group after 3 months:

Table 4.12 & Figure 4.9 shows the anthropometric parameters for 6 weeks DYP group pre and post Yoga. No significant change was found between weight (mean ± SD = 70.25 ± 11.93 to 70.44 ± 12.27,p-0.749), BMI (mean ± SD = 29.81 ± 4.88 to 29.17± 4.94,p-0.771), WC (mean ± SD = 93.89± 10.11 to 91.73 ± 11.80, p-0.061), HC (mean ± SD = 104.43 ± 11.54 to 103.46 ± 11.36, p-0.383) and WHR (mean ± SD = 0.90 ± 0.07 to 0.89 ± 0.06,p-0.280) after 6 weeks of Yoga. Moreover, Table 4.13 & Figure 4.9 shows the anthropometric parameters for 12 weeks DYP group pre and post Yoga. Significant decrease was found between weight (mean ± SD

= 68.32±9.89 to 66.88 ±9.88 p-< 0.001), BMI (mean ± SD = 28.32±3.89 to 27.72 ± 3.87,p< 0.001), WC (mean± SD =93.15 ±8.37 to 91.40 ±9.20, p-0.041) and HC (mean ± SD = 103.85±8.47 to 101.63±8.68 p-0.018) in 12 weeks DYP group, However WHR did not change significantly (mean ± SD = 0.90±0.06 to 0.90± 0.05,p=0.897) in the 12 weeks DYP group.

Discussion of the results:

The anthropometric parameters show no significant changes in 6 weeks DYP group whereas all the anthropometric parameters in 12 weeks DYP group show significant improvements except WHR. The results of the present study highlight the importance of adherence based long-term duration of the Yoga intervention on anthropometric parameters. The comprehensive discussion of the same section has been also mentioned on section 4.1.2.

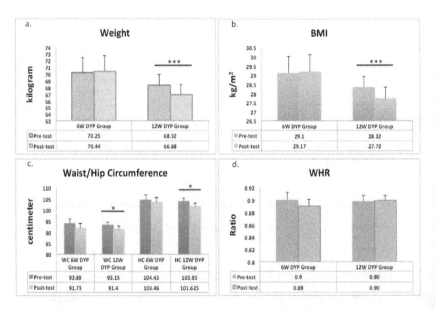

Figure 4.9 a) Mean changes in weight for pre-test and post-test for 6 weeks and 12 weeks DYP group *(p< 0.001***)* **b)** Mean changes in BMI for pre and post test for 6 weeks and 12 weeks DYP group *(p< 0.001***)* **c)** Mean changes in WC and HC for pre and post test for 6 weeks and 12 weeks DYP group *(p< .041*, p< .018*)* **d)**Mean difference of WHR for pre and post test for 6 weeks and 12 weeks DYP group.

Table 4.13: Pre-Post comparison in selected anthropometric parameters like weight, BMI, WC, HC and WHR in Mean, SD and Mean difference, t-value with p- values at Pre-test and Post-test in 12 weeks DYP group.

Anthropometric Parameters	Test Condition	Mean	SD	95% CI		t-value	p-value
				Lower	Upper		
Weight	Pre test	68.32	9.89	0.76	2.12	4.28	**< 0.001**
	Post test	66.88	9.88				
BMI	Pre test	28.32	3.89	0.32	0.89	4.27	**< 0.001**
	Post test	27.72	3.87				
WC	Pre test	93.15	8.37	0.08	3.42	2.12	**.041**
	Post test	91.40	9.20				
HC	Pre test	103.85	8.47	0.41	4.04	2.48	**.018**
	Post test	101.63	8.68				
WHR	Pre test	0.90	0.06	-0.02	0.02	-0.13	0.897
	Post test	0.90	0.05				

Data expressed in Mean, SD, and statistical significance (*p< 0.001**, p< .041*, p< .018**) BMI- Body Mass Index, WC-Waist Circumference, HC- Hip Circumference, WHR- Waist Hip Ratio, SD= Standard Deviation, CI- Confidence Interval, DYP- Diabetic Yoga Protocol.

Table 4.14: Pre-Post test mean comparison in selected neuropsychological parameters viz. sustained attention, general health, state anxiety, perceived stress in mean, SD and t-value with p- values at pre test and post test in 6 weeks DYP group.

Neuropsychological parameters	Test Condition	Mean	SD	95% CI		t-value	p-value
				Lower	Upper		
Sustained Attention	Pre test	24.00	10.23	-10.84	-4.20	-4.68	< 0.001
	Post test	31.52	11.16				
General Health	Pre test	15.48	4.34	3.81	8.67	5.30	< 0.001
	Post test	9.24	3.96				
State Anxiety	Pre test	46.68	11.75	8.69	19.63	5.35	< 0.001
	Post test	32.52	9.89				
Perceived Stress	Pre test	21.00	4.78	5.23	9.55	7.02	< 0.001
	Post test	13.61	4.35				

Data expressed in mean, SD, and statistical significance (*p< 0.001****) SD= Standard Deviation, CI=Confidence Interval.

4.1.9 Comparison of the Pre-test and Post-test difference neuropsychological parameters in the 6 weeks DYP group and 12 weeks DYP group after 3 months:

Table 4.14 and Figure 4.10 indicate the mean difference between various neuropsychological parameters in 6 weeks DYP group. Score of various tests significantly improved after performing Yoga for 6 weeks. Sustained attention score increased significantly from 24.00 ± 10.23 to 31.52 ± 11.16 (p< 0.001), general health decreased from 15.48 ± 4.34 to 9.24 ± 3.96 (p< 0.001), state anxiety decreased from 46.68 ±11.75 to 32.52 ± 9.89 (p< 0.001) and perceived stress also decreased significantly from 21.00 ± 4.78 to 13.61 ± 4.35 (p< 0.001). Table 4.15 & Figure 4.10 indicate the mean difference between various neuropsychological parameters in 12 weeks DYP group. Score of various tests significantly improved after performing DYP for 12 weeks. Sustained attention score (mean± SD = 23.89±10.09 to 28.85±10.90, p= 0.003) increased significantly whereas general health (mean ±SD = 13.70±3.87 to 7.41±2.47, p< 0.001), state anxiety (mean ± SD = 45.41±8.35 to

102

31.19±6.32 p< 0.001) and perceived stress scores decreased significantly (mean ± SD
= 18.70±7.34 to 13.03±5.28, p< 0.001).

Discussion of the results:

Neuropsychological parameters like sustained attention, general health, state anxiety
and perceived stress shown significant improvement in both the intervention groups
like 6 weeks DYP and 12 weeks DYP group. The beneficial effect of Yoga on
neuropsychological and cognitive functions was well documented in the previous
literature. The present study also suggests that both the long term and short term
practices bring positive changes in overall mood and behavior. The comprehensive
discussion of the same section has been also mentioned on section 4.1.3

Table 4.15: Pre- Post comparison in selected neuropsychological parameters viz.
sustained attention, general health, state anxiety, perceived stress in mean, SD and
mean difference and t-value with p- values at pre-test and post-test in 12 weeks DYP
group.

Neuropsychological parameters	Test Condition	Mean	SD	95% CI		t-value	p-value
				Lower	Upper		
Sustained	Pre test	23.89	10.09	-8.11	-1.82	-3.24	**0.003**
Attention	Post test	28.85	10.90				
General	Pre test	13.70	3.87	4.83	7.76	8.85	**< 0.001**
Health	Post test	7.41	2.47				
State	Pre test	45.41	8.35	11.18	17.27	9.61	**< 0.001**
Anxiety	Post test	31.19	6.32				
Perceived	Pre test	18.70	7.34	3.04	8.31	4.35	**< 0.001**
Stress	Post test	13.03	5.28				

Data expressed in Mean, SD, and atatistical significance *(p< 0.001***, p< .003**)*,
SD= Standard Deviation, CI- Confidence Interval.

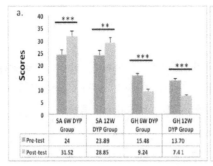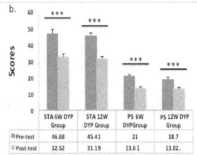

Figure 4.10:(a) SA denotes Sustained attention; GH denotes General health; Mean changes in sustained attention and General health for pre-test and post-test for 6 weeks *(p< 0.001***)* and 12 weeks DYP group *(p< 0.003**, p< 0.001***)* b) STA denotes State anxiety ; PS denotes Perceived stress ; Mean changes in State anxiety and Perceived stress for pre and post test for 6 weeks *(p< 0.001***)* and 12 weeks DYP group *(p< 0.001***)*

Table 4.16: Pre-Post comparison in selected Molecular markers like Angiogenin, VEGF and BDNF in Mean, SD and t-values with p- values at pre-test and post-test in 6 weeks DYP Group.

Molecular Markers	Test Condition	Mean	SD	95% CI		t-value	p-value
				Lower	Upper		
Angiogenin	Pre test	0.704	0.823	-0.723	-0.021	-2.172	**0.039**
	Post test	1.076	1.298				
VEGF	Pre test	0.0132	0.010	-0.005	0.001	-1.385	0.177
	Post test	0.0154	0.013				
BDNF	Pre test	73.53	130.37	-49.725	36.120	-0.325	0.748
	Post test	80.33	188.61				

Data expressed in mean, SD, and statistical significance *(p<0.039*)* VEGF- Vascular Endothelial Growth; BDNF- Brain Derived Neurotropic Factor, SD= Standard Deviation, Diff-Difference, CI- Confidence Interval, DYP- Diabetic Yoga Protocol.

4.1.10 Comparison of the Pre-test and Post-test difference of molecular markers in the 6 weeks DYP group and 12 weeks DYP group after 3 months:

Table 4.16 & Figure 4.11 shows the difference between various protein levels in the individuals after performing Yoga for 6 weeks. Angiogenin (mean ± SD =0.704 ±0.823 to 1.076±1.298) increased significantly in the post group. (p-0.039). No significant difference was found between protein levels of VEGF (mean ± SD = 0.0132±0.010 to 0.0154± 0.013,p-0.177) and BDNF (mean ± SD = 73.53±130.37 to 80.33±188.61,p-0.748). Moreover, Table 4.17 & Figure 4.11 shows the difference between various protein levels in the individuals after performing Yoga for 12 weeks. No significant difference was found between protein levels of ANG (mean ± SD = 0.461± 0.561to0.525 ±0.590, p=0.414), VEGF (mean ± SD = 0.0143±0.012 to 0.0159±0.011, p=0.150) and BDNF (mean ± SD = 43.50± 50.48to 42.04±43.62, p=0.862).

Discussion of the results:

The angiogenin levels were significantly improved in 6W DYP whereas other parameters (VEGF & BDNF) didn't show significant changes. Likewise, results shown in 12 weeks DYP group where no significant changes were seen on either of the selected molecular markers. However, improvement in mean was seen in selected molecular markers but not at significant level. The result on molecular markers suggest the need of continuation of Yogic practices for longer period of time in an adherent way. The comprehensive discussion of the same section has been also mentioned on section 4.1.4

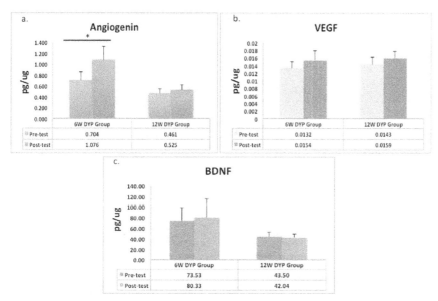

Figure 4.11(a) Mean changes in angiogenin for pre-test and post-test for 6 weeks *(p< .039*)* and 12 weeks DYP group *(p< 0.001***)* **b)** Mean changes in VEGF for pre and post test for 6 weeks and 12 weeks DYP group **c)** Mean changes in BDNF for pre and post test for 6 weeks and 12 weeks DYP group.

Table 4.17: Pre-Post test mean comparison in selected molecular markers like angiogenin, VEGF and BDNF in mean, SD and t-values with p- values at pre-test and post-test in 12 weeks DYP Group.

Molecular Markers	Test Condition	Mean	SD	95% CI		t-value	p-value
				Lower	Upper		
Angiogenin	Pre test	0.461	0.561	-0.221	0.093	-0.83	0.414
	Post test	0.525	0.590				
VEGF	Pre test	0.0143	0.012	-0.004	0.001	-1.47	0.150
	Post test	0.0159	0.011				
BDNF	Pre test	43.50	50.48	-15.433	18.354	0.18	0.862
	Post test	42.04	43.62				

Data expressed in Mean, SD, and statistical significance ANG- Angiogenin; VEGF- Vascular Endothelial Growth; BDNF- Brain Derived Neurotropic Factor, SD= Standard Deviation, CI- Confidence Interval, DYP- Diabetic Yoga Protocol.

Table 4.18: Pre-post test mean comparison in selected Hormonal markers i.e. Cortisol and Leptin in mean, SD and t-value with p- values at Pre-test and Post-test in 6 weeks DYP and 12 weeks DYP group.

Hormonal Markers	Test Condition	Mean	SD	95% CI		t-value	p-value
				Lower	Upper		
Cortisol 6W DYP	Pre test	0.00127	0.00115	-0.00119	0.00013	-1.66	0.109
	Post test	0.00180	0.00141				
Leptin 6W DYP	Pre test	0.00027	0.00012	-0.00009	0.00006	-0.43	0.672
	Post test	0.00028	0.00022				
Cortisol 12W DYP	Pre test	0.00108	0.00110	-0.00103	0.00011	-1.62	0.113
	Post test	0.00154	0.00148				
Leptin 12W DYP	Pre test	0.00028	0.00033	-0.00008	0.00003	-0.82	0.418
	Post test	0.00030	0.00029				

Data expressed in Mean, SD, and Statistical significance SD= Standard Deviation, CI- Confidence Interval, DYP- Diabetic Yoga Protocol.

4.1.11 Comparison of the Pre-test and Post-test difference of Hormonal markers in the 6 weeks DYP group and 12 weeks DYP group after 3 months:

Table 4.18 & Figure 4.12 indicates the mean difference between levels of leptin and cortisol hormones for 6 weeks DYP and 12 weeks DYP group. No significant difference was there between levels of both hormones [leptin (mean ± SD = 0.00027± 0.00012 to 0.00028±0.00022,p-0.672), cortisol (mean ± SD = 0.00127±0.00115 to 0.00180±0.00141,p=0.109) at 6 weeks and 12 weeks [leptin (mean ± SD = 0.00028±0.00033to 0.00030±0.00029,p=0.418), cortisol (mean ± SD = 0.00108±0.00110 to 0.00154±0.00148, p=0.113) time points.

Discussion of the results:

The leptin and cortisol levels didn't show significant changes in 6W DYP group and 12W DYP group. The result on hormonal markers suggests the need of continuation of Yogic practices for longer period of time in an adherent way. The comprehensive discussion of the same section has been also mentioned on section 4.1.5

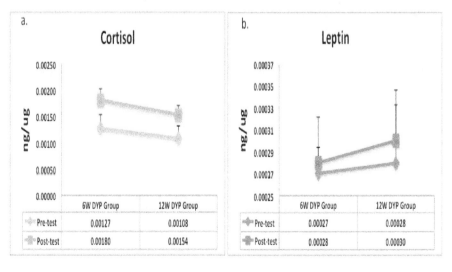

Figure 4.12 a) Mean changes in Cortisol levels for pre-test and post-test for 6 weeks and 12 weeks DYP group; Cortisol (ng/ug)- ng of cortisol in ug of total protein**b)** Mean changes in Leptin levels between pre and post test for 6 weeks and 12 weeks DYP group *(p<0 .038*);* Leptin (ng/ug)- ng of leptin in ug of total protein.

Table 4.19: Pre-Post test mean comparison 6 weeks DYP at pre-test and post-test on various domains of QoL i.e. Physical, Psychological, Social and Environmental domain along with overall QoL in mean, SD, mean difference, and t- value with p-values at pre-test and Post-test in 6 weeks DYP group.

Domains of QoL	Test Condition	Mean	SD	95% CI		t-value	p-value
				Lower	Upper		
Physical Domain	Pre test	56.96	8.89	-8.63	-0.49	-2.31	**0.030**
	Post test	61.52	8.52				
Psychological Domain	Pre test	56.32	7.73	-7.61	4.81	-0.47	0.646
	Post test	57.72	11.83				
Social Domain	Pre test	65.8	12.54	-13.32	-3.64	-3.62	**0.001**
	Post test	74.28	15.05				
Environmental Domain	Pre test	73.2	9.46	-14.46	-4.42	-3.88	**0.001**
	Post test	82.64	11.03				
QoL	Pre test	251.96	23.77	-37.61	-15.27	-4.89	**< 0.001**
	Post test	278.40	33.25				

Data expressed in Mean, SD, and Statistical significance(**p= 0.030*,p=001**, p< 0.001)** SD= Standard Deviation, CI- Confidence Interval, DYP- Diabetic Yoga Protocol

4.1.12 Comparison of the pre-test and post-test difference of Overall QOL and domains of QOL in the 6 weeks DYP group and 12 weeks DYP group after 3 months:

The QoL increased significantly after performing Yoga for 6 weeks from pre-test 251.96±23.77 (mean±SD) to post 278.40±33.25 (mean±SD) with p< 0.001(Table 4.19 & Figure 4.13). Significant increase was found in physical (mean ± SD = 56.96± 8.89 to 61.52±8.52 (p< 0.030), social (mean ± SD = 65.8± 12.54 to 74.28±15.05, p<0.001) and environmental (mean ± SD =73.2 ± 9.46to 82.64±11.03, p<0.001) domains of QoL as shown in Table 4.20 and Figure 4.13 (p-values: 0.030, 0.001 and 0.001 respectively). However, Psychological domain reported no significant changes with p< 0.646).

Similarly, in twelve weeks the QoL increased significantly from pre-test 246.14±27.76 (mean±SD) to post 290.29±38.38 (mean±SD) with p-value- **p< 0.001** (Table 4.20 & Figure 4.14). Significant increase was found in physical (mean ± SD =

108

55.00±9.62 **to** 61.74±8.49), psychological (mean ± SD =55.59 ± 8.02 to65.37±11.70), social (mean ± SD = 62.26±16.51to78.04 ±12.89) and environmental (mean ± SD = 73.30±8.09 **to** 84.85± 84.85) domains of QoL as shown in Table 4.21 & Figure 4.14 (p-values: **0.005,p< 0.001, p< 0.001, p< 0.001**) respectively.

Discussion of the results :

Overall QoL and its associated domains show significant improvements in both the 6W DYP and 12W DYP groups except psychological domain in 6W DYP group. For instance, the non significant changes in the psychological domain in 6W DYP group and significant changes in 12W DYP group demonstrated that psychological domain might be affected by the duration of DYP.. Furthermore, the result shows that either short term or long term Yogic and meditative practices bring significant improvements in overall QoL. The comprehensive discussion of the same section has been also mentioned on section 4.1.6

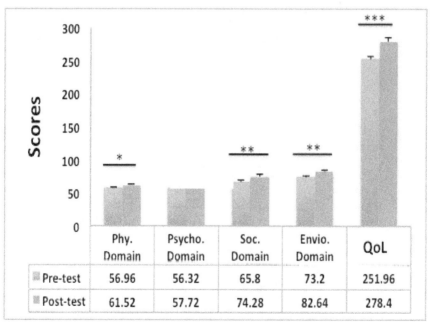

Figure 4.13 The mean change in levels of Overall QoL and its domains at pre DYP and post DYP in 6 weeks DYP group with statistical significance (*p< 0.030*, p< .001**, p< 0.001*), Phy -Physical domain, Psycho - Psychological domain, Socio-Social domain and Enviro- Environmental domain.

Table 4.20: Mean comparison in 12 weeks DYP group at pre-test and post-test on various domains of Quality of life i.e Physical, Psychological, Social and Environmental domain along with QoL in mean, SD, mean difference, and t- value with p- values at pre-test and Post-test in 12 weeks DYP group.

Domains of QoL	Test Condition	Mean	SD	95% CI Lower	95% CI Upper	t-value	p-value
Physical Domain	Pre test	55.00	9.62	-11.28	-2.21	-3.06	**0.005**
	Post test	61.74	8.49				
Psychological Domain	Pre test	55.59	8.02	-14.57	-4.99	-4.20	**< 0.001**
	Post test	65.37	11.70				
Social Domain	Pre test	62.26	16.51	-23.78	-7.78	-4.05	**< 0.001**
	Post test	78.04	12.89				
Environmental Domain	Pre test	73.30	8.09	-16.55	-6.56	-4.76	**< 0.001**
	Post test	84.85	14.75				
QoL	Pre test	246.15	27.77	-59.10	-29.19	-6.07	**< 0.001**
	Post test	290.30	38.38				

Data expressed in mean, SD, and statistical significance (p= 0.005**, *p< 0.001***)*
SD= Standard Deviation, CI- Confidence Interval, DYP- Diabetic Yoga Protocol

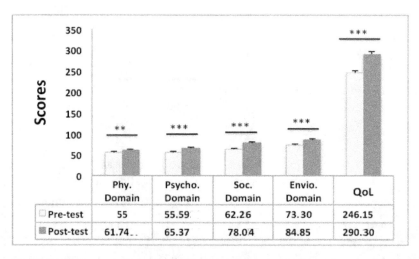

Figure 4.14 The mean change in levels of Overall QoL and its domains at pre DYP and post DYP in 12 weeks DYP group with statistical significance*(p< 0.005**, p< 0.001***).*Phy -Physical domain, Psycho - Psychological domain, Socio- Social domain and Enviro- Environmental domain.

110

4.2 GROUP WISE DIFFERENCES AMONG CONTROL, 6W (6 WEEKS) DYP AND 12W (12 WEEKS) DYP GROUP:

The one-way ANOVA test was used to for determining the differences between three groups. The analysis for control and DYP group was analyzed earlier. We further divided the section of our present study according to the attendance of the participants and on the basis of that between the DYP group we divided the participants further in two categories according to their presence at the Yoga classes. The DYP group was divided into 6 weeks DYP group and 12 weeks DYP group. So, the analysis among Control, 6 weeks DYP group and 12 weeks DYP group were discussed

Table 4.21: Analysis of variance (ANOVA) among control, 6 weeks DYP group and 12 weeks DYP group in selected biochemical parameters i.e HbA1c and FBG in mean, sum of squares, mean squares and F ratio with p- values.

Variables		Group Mean			Source of Variance	Sum of Squares	df	Mean Squares	F-Value	P-Value
		6 weeks	12 weeks	Control Group						
HbA1c	Pre test	5.6	5.67	5.87	Between Groups	1.31	2	0.65	2.189	0.118
					Within Groups	28.05	94	0.30		
	Post test	5.47	5.57	5.72	Between Groups	0.98	2	0.49	1.810	0.169
					Within Groups	25.55	94	0.27		
FBG	Pre Test	90.55	100.34	96.81	Between Groups	1488.76	2	744.38	2.903	0.060
					Within Groups	24105.30	94	256.44		
	Post Test	98.64	102.33	96.87	Between Groups	543.50	2	271.75	0.725	0.487
					Within Groups	35235.60	94	374.85		

Data expressed in mean, sum of squares, mean squares, F value and statistical significance, HbA1c – Glycated Haemoglobin; FBG- Fasting Blood Glucose, df- degree of freedom, DYP- Diabetic Yoga Protocol

4.2.1 Comparison of the group wise differences among control, 6 weeks and 12 weeks DYP group on biochemical parameters:

The mean pre-test value for HbA1c (Table 4.21) for 6 weeks and 12 weeks and control group was 5.6, 5.67 and 5.87 respectively. The obtained F ratio for sum of squares and mean squares was calculated as 2.189 (p= 0.118). Therefore, pre-test was not significant (p>0.05). Hence, there is no significant difference between groups for the pre-test on HbA1c levels. The mean HbA1c values for post test was 5.47, 5.57, 5.72 for 6 weeks and 12 weeks DYP and control group respectively. The obtained "F" ratio was 1.810 (p=0.169), which was insignificant (p>0.05). Thus, there is non-significant difference between groups for HbA1c post-test as shown in Figure 4.15 (a).

Furthermore, the average scores for Pre-test FBG for 6 weeks, 12 weeks and control group were 90.55, 100.34 and 96.81 respectively. The obtained F value was 2.903 and p value were 0.060, which was statistically insignificant among, 6 weeks, 12 weeks and control group. Similarly, the post -test FBG also shows no significant differences among three groups (control-98.64,6 weeks-102.33, 12 weeks-96.87) with F ratio of 0.725 and p value of 0.487 as shown in Figure 4.15 (b).

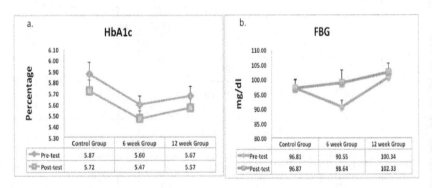

Figure 4.15: a) Mean difference between HbA1c levels for pre-test and post-test among Control group ,6 weeks and 12 weeks DYP group. **b)** Mean difference between FBG for pre-test and post-test among Control group , 6 weeks and 12 weeks DYP group.

Table 4.22: Pre- post analysis of variance among control, 6 weeks DYP group and 12 weeks DYP group in selected Anthropometric parameters like weight, BMI, WC, HC and WHR in mean, sum of squares, mean squares and F ratio with p- values.

Variables		6 weeks DYP	12 weeks DYP	Control Group	Source of Variance	Sum of Squares	df	Mean Squares	F-Value	P-Value
		Group Mean								
Weight	Pre test	70.25	68.32	71.62	Between Groups	203.3	2	101.65	0.726	0.487
					Within Groups	13865.84	99	140.06		
	Post test	70.44	66.88	70.86	Between Groups	352.08	2	176.04	1.263	0.287
					Within Groups	13798.68	99	139.38		
BMI	Pre Test	29.10	28.32	29.57	Between Groups	29.71	2	14.86	0.721	0.489
					Within Groups	2041.04	99	20.62		
	Post Test	29.17	27.72	29.27	Between Groups	55.77	2	27.89	1.354	0.263
					Within Groups	2039.55	99	20.60		
WC	Pre test	93.89	93.15	96.39	Between Groups	200.88	2	100.44	0.906	0.408
					Within Groups	10869.66	98	110.92		
	Post test	91.73	91.40	97.51	Between Groups	811.83	2	405.91	3.493	**0.034**
					Within Groups	11504.58	99	116.21		
HC	Pre test	104.43	103.85	103.94	Between Groups	6.00	2	3.00	0.026	0.974
					Within Groups	11421.84	99	115.37		
	Post test	103.46	101.63	105.68	Between Groups	301.68	2	150.84	1.442	0.241
					Within Groups	10356.28	99	104.61		
WHR	Pre test	0.90	0.90	0.93	Between Groups	0.02	2	0.009	2.713	0.071
					Within Groups	0.34	98	0.003		
	Post test	0.89	0.90	0.92	Between Groups	0.02	2	0.010	3.021	0.053
					Within Groups	0.32	98	0.003		

Data expressed in mean, sum of squares, Mean squares, F value and statistical significance (p< .034*), BMI – Body Mass Index; WC- Waist Circumference; HC- Hip Circumference; WHR-Waist Hip Ratio, df- degree of freedom, DYP- Diabetic Yoga Protocol

4.2.2   Comparison of the group wise differences among control 6 weeks and 12 weeks DYP group on Anthropometric parameters:

The pre-test mean values for 6 weeks, 12 weeks and control group (Table-4.22) with regard to weight were 70.25, 68.32 and 71.62 respectively. No significant differences were found between three groups with F ratio of 0.726 and p value of 0.487. Similar results were obtained after post – test among three groups (6 weeks=70.44, 12 weeks=66.88, control=70.86) with F value of 1.263 and p value of 0.287. Hence, statistically non –significant differences was found between three groups on weight as shown in Figure 4.16 (a).

Furthermore, no statistical significant differences were seen between 6 weeks DYP, 12 weeks DYP and control group at pre-test (F ratio- .721, P=0.489) as well as post –test (F ratio=1.354, P=0.263) level for BMI as shown in Figure 4.16 (b). Likewise, the Pre- test WC shows no significant (p=0.408) difference between 6 weeks DYP (Mean-93.89), 12 weeks DYP (Mean- 93.15) and control group (Mean-96.39) with F ratio of 0.906. However, the statistically significant differences was seen between three groups (6 weeks DYP-91.73, 12 weeks DYP- 91.40, Control-97.51) on WC after post-test with F ratio of 3.493 (**p< .034**) as shown in Figure 4.16(c).

Moreover, pre-test HC values between 6 weeks DYP (104.43), 12 weeks DYP (103.85) and control group (103.94) shows no significant (p=0.974) differences with F ratio of .026. Similar results was seen after post test on HC values between three groups (6 weeks DYP-103.46, 12 weeks DYP-101.61, Control-105.68) with the obtained F ratio of 1.442 and p value of 0.241 which was found to be statistically insignificant as shown in Figure 4.16 (c).

Besides, WHR shows no statistically significant differences between 6 weeks DYP, 12 weeks DYP and control group on either of the levels i.e. pre-test (F ratio=2.713, p=0.071) and post-test (F ratio-3.021,p=.053)as shown in Figure 4.16 (d).

114

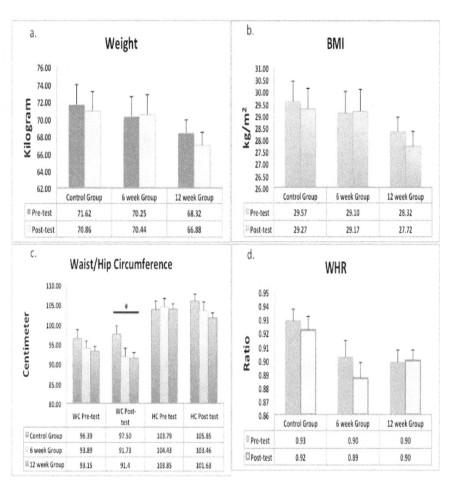

Figure 4.16: a) Mean difference between weight for pre-test and post-test among Control group , 6 weeks and 12 weeks DYP group. **b)** Mean difference between BMI for pre-test and post-test among Control group , 6 weeks and 12 weeks DYP group. **c)** Mean difference between Waist/Hip circumference for pre-test and post-test among control group , 6 weeks and 12 weeks DYP group*(p< 0.034 *)*,**d)** Mean difference between WHR for pre-test and post-test among Control group , 6 weeks and 12 weeks DYP group.

Table 4.23: Analysis of variance among control , 6 weeks DYP group and 12 weeks DYP group in selected neuropsychological parameters like sustained attention, general health, state anxiety and perceived stress in mean, sum of squares , mean squares and F ratio with p- values.

Variables		Group Mean			Source of Variance	Sum of Squares	df	Mean Squares	F-Value	P-Value
		6 weeks	12 weeks	Control Group						
Sustained Attention	Pre test	24	23.89	21.8	Between Groups	66.45	2	33.23	0.309	0.735
					Within Groups	7427.87	69	107.65		
	Post test	31.52	28.85	24.2	Between Groups	601.14	2	300.57	2.088	0.132
					Within Groups	9932.85	69	143.95		
General Health	Pre Test	15.48	13.7	13.65	Between Groups	52.86	2	26.43	1.841	0.166
					Within Groups	990.42	69	14.35		
	Post Test	9.24	7.41	12.45	Between Groups	293.75	2	146.88	15.639	< 0.001
					Within Groups	648.03	69	9.39		
State Anxiety	Pre Test	46.68	45.41	42.2	Between Groups	231.72	2	115.86	1.044	0.357
					Within Groups	7655.16	69	110.94		
	Post Test	32.52	31.19	36.6	Between Groups	352.21	2	176.10	2.268	0.111
					Within Groups	5357.11	69	77.64		
Perceived Stress	Pre Test	21	18.7	18.91	Between Groups	99.38	2	49.69	1.323	0.271
					Within Groups	3719.14	99	37.57		
	Post Test	13.61	13.02	17.26	Between Groups	368.25	2	184.12	5.47	0.006
					Within Groups	3332.27	99	33.66		

Data expressed in mean, sum of squares, mean squares, F value and statistical significance *(p< 0.001***, p< .006*)*, df- degree of freedom, DYP- Diabetic Yoga Protocol

4.2.3 Comparison of the group wise differences among control 6 weeks and 12 weeks DYP group on neuropsychological parameters:

Table 4.23 showing analysis of variances for selected neuropsychological parameters i.e sustained attention, general health, state anxiety and perceived stress among 6 weeks DYP group, 12 weeks DYP group and control group. The means scores at the pre- test for sustained attention were 24.0, 23.89 and 21.80 for 6 weeks, 12 weeks and control group respectively. The "F" ratio of pre –test sustained attention levels was found to be 0.309 (p=0.735) which is not significant (p>0.05) at 5% level of significance. Likewise, the post test result of sustained attention also shows no significant results between three groups (6 weeks-31.25, 12 weeks-28.85, Control-24.40 with "F" ratio of 2.088 (p=0.132) as shown in Figure 4.17(a)

Additionally, the mean pre test general health levels for 6 weeks, 12 weeks and control group were 15.48,13.70 and 13.65 respectively. The "F ratio" was determined as 1.841 with p value of 0.166. Thus, no significant differences (p>0.05) were found between the groups. The post-test GHQ levels reveals the mean values of 9.24 for 6 weeks, 7.41 for 12 weeks, 12.45 for control group. The calculated "F" ratio was 15.639 shows statistically significant difference (p< 0.001) for general health levels for post-test between the groups as shown in figure 4.17(a). The state anxiety values for pre-test (6 weeks DYP -46.68, 12 weeks DYP -45.41, control-42.20) and post-test (6 weeks DYP -32.52, 12 weeks DYP -31.19, control-36.60) shows no significant differences between groups. The obtained "F" ratio for state anxiety pre-test and post –test was 1.044 and 2.268 respectively. However, the p values for state anxiety pre and post test was 0.357 and 0.111 which was not significant as shown in Figure 4.17(b).

Moreover, the pre-test mean scores for perceived stress were 21.0 for 6 weeks, 18.70 for 12 weeks and 18.91 for control group with F ratio of 1.323 and p value of 0.271, which was non-significant. Though, post-test perceived stress levels shows statistically significant (p< .006) differences between 6 weeks DYP group (13.61), 12 weeks DYP (13.02) group and control (17.26) group with F ratio of 5.470 as shown in Figure 4.17(b).

117

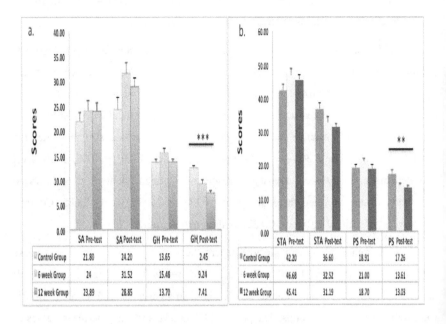

Figure 4.17: a) Mean difference of sustained attention and general health for pre-test and post-test among control group , 6 weeks and 12 weeks DYP group.*(p<0.001***);* SA denotes Sustained attention; GH denotes General health **b)** Mean difference between state anxiety and perceived stress for pre-test and post-test among control group , 6 weeks and 12 weeks DYP group *(p< .006*);* STA denotes State anxiety ; PS denotes Perceived stress.

Table 4.24: Pre-post Analysis of variance among control, 6 weeks DYP group and 12 weeks DYP group in selected molecular markers i.e angiogenin ,VEGF and BDNF in mean, sum of squares , mean squares and F ratio with p- values.

Variables		Group Mean			Source of Variance	Sum of Squares	df	Mean Squares	F-Value	P-Value
		6 weeks	12 weeks	Control Group						
Angiogenin	Pre test	0.70	0.46	6.80	Between Groups	882.43	2	441.22	12.076	< 0.001
					Within Groups	3616.99	99	36.54		
	Post test	1.08	0.53	5.51	Between Groups	518.29	2	259.15	12.419	< 0.001
					Within Groups	2065.77	99	20.87		
VEGF	Pre Test	0.013	0.014	0.022	Between Groups	0.002	2	0.001	5.616	0.005
					Within Groups	0.014	97	0.000		
	Post Test	0.015	0.016	0.016	Between Groups	0.000	2	0.000	0.047	0.954
					Within Groups	0.011	97	0.000		
BDNF	Pre Test	73.53	43.50	34.97	Between Groups	24657.84	2	12328.92	1.988	0.143
					Within Groups	595439.89	96	6202.50		
	Post Test	80.33	42.04	25.94	Between Groups	47091.71	2	23545.85	2.105	0.127
					Within Groups	1073627.67	96	11183.62		

Data expressed in Mean, Sum of squares, Mean squares, F value and Statistical significance *(p< 0.001***, p< .005**)* VEGF- Vascular Endothelial Growth Factor; BDNF-Brain Derived Neurotropic factor, df- degree of freedom, DYP- Diabetic Yoga Protocol.

4.2.4 Comparison of the group wise differences among control, 6 weeks and 12 weeks DYP group on molecular markers:

Table 4.24 showing analysis of variances for selected molecular markers i.e Angiogenin, VEGF and BDNF among 6 weeks DYP group, 12 weeks DYP group and control group. The selected molecular markers for the present were Angiogenin, VEGF and BDNF. The Angiogenin levels in the study found to be statistically significant at both pre-test (6 weeks DYP -0.70,12 weeks DYP -0.46, Control group- 6.80) and post –test (6 weeks DYP -1.08, 12 weeks DYP - 0.53, Control group- 5.51) levels between 6 weeks DYP group, 12 weeks DYP group and control group. The angiogenin pre –test F value was 12.076 with $p < 0.001$ value and post test F value was with $p < 0.001$ as shown in Figure 4.18 (a). Furthermore, the VEGF levels for pre-test 6 weeks group, 12 weeks DYP group and control group were .0132042, .0143015 and .0221771 respectively. The obtained F ratio for Pre-test VEGF levels was 5.616 with $p < .005$ which was found to be statistically significant as shown in Figure 4.11 (b).Hence, there is a statistically significant difference found between 6 weeks DYP group, 12 weeks DYP group and control group. But, no significant difference was observed after post-test between 6 weeks DYP group, 12 weeks DYP group and control group with F ratio of .047 and p value of .954 as shown in Figure 4.18 (b) In addition, the BDNF levels shows non-significant differences at both the levels i.e pre-test and post-test between 6 weeks DYP group, 12 weeks DYP group and control group with pre-test F ratio of 1.988 and post-test F ratio of 2.105. The pre-test p value was 0.143 and post-test p value is 0.127, which was found to be statistically insignificant as shown in Figure 4.18 (c).

.

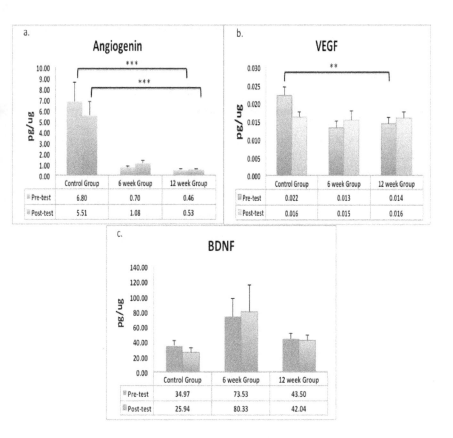

Figure 4.18: a) Mean difference between Angiogenin for pre-test and post-test among control group , 6 weeks and 12 weeks DYP group*(p< 0.001***)*. **b)** Mean difference on VEGF for pre-test and post-test among Control group , 6 weeks and 12 weeks DYP group. **c)** Mean difference on BDNF for pre-test and post-test among Control group , 6 weeks and 12 weeks DYP group(*p<0.005**).*

Table 4.25: Analysis of variance between control, 6 weeks DYP group and 12 weeks DYP group in selected Hormonal markers i.e Cortisol and Leptin in mean, sum of squares , mean squares and F ratio with p- values.

Variables		6 weeks	12 weeks	Control Group	Source of Variance	Sum of Squares	df	Mean Squares	F-Ratio	P-Value
Cortisol	Pre test	0.0013	0.0011	0.0017	Between Groups	0.000	2	0.000	2.08	0.13
					Within Groups	0.000	99	0.000		
	Post test	0.0018	0.0015	0.0012	Between Groups	0.000	2	0.000	1.304	0.276
					Within Groups	0.000	99	0.000		
Leptin	Pre Test	0.00027	0.00028	0.00044	Between Groups	0.000	2	0.000	3.742	**0.027**
					Within Groups	0.000	99	0.000		
	Post Test	0.00028	0.00030	0.00042	Between Groups	0.000	2	0.000	2.131	0.124
					Within Groups	0.000	99	0.000		

Data expressed in mean, sum of squares, mean squares, F value and statistical significance *(p< 0.027*)*, df- degree of freedom, DYP- Diabetic Yoga Protocol

4.2.5 Comparison of the group wise differences among control 6 weeks and 12 weeks DYP group on hormonal markers:

Table 4.25 showing analysis of variances for selected hormonal markers i.e Cortisol and Leptin among 6 weeks DYP group, 12 weeks DYP group and control group. The mean cortisol values for Pre-test in 6 weeks DYP group, 12 weeks DYP group and control group were 0.0013, 0.0011 and 0.0017 respectively. The pre-test cortisol levels F ratio was 2.080 and p value were 0.130, which was found to be statistically insignificant. Hence, there is no significant differences were found between groups at pre-test level. Likewise, results was obtained after post-test for cortisol levels with F ratio of 1.304 and p value of 0.276 which was also found to be non-significant as shown in Figure 4.19 (a).

Additionally, the pre-test leptin levels shows statistically significant (p<. **027**) differences between 6 weeks DYP group (0.00027), 12 weeks DYP (0.00028) group and control (0.00044) group with F ratio of 3.742 as shown in Figure 4.12(b). But, no significant difference was seen after post-test between 6 weeks DYP group (0.00028), 12 weeks DYP (0.00030) group and control (0.00042) group on leptin levels. The obtained post-test F ratio for leptin levels were 2.131 with p value .124 as shown in Figure 4.19 (b).

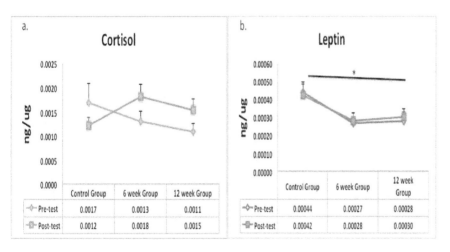

Figure 4.19: a) Mean difference between cortisol for pre-test and post-test among Control group , 6 weeks and 12 weeks DYP group. **b)** Mean difference on Leptin for pre-test and post-test among control group , 6 weeks and 12 weeks DYP group *(p <0. 027)*

Table 4.26: Analysis of variance between control, 6 weeks DYP group and 12 weeks DYP group on various domains of QoL i.e. physical, psychological, social and environmental in mean, sum of squares, mean squares and F ratio with p- values.

Variables		6 weeks	12 weeks	Control Group	Source of Variance	Sum of Squares	df	Mean Squares	F-Value	P-Value
		Group Mean								
Physical Domain	Pre test	56.96	55.00	57.90	Between Groups	105.23	2	52.61	0.690	0.505
					Within Groups	5260.76	69	76.24		
	Post test	61.52	61.74	57.60	Between Groups	235.76	2	117.88	1.785	0.175
					Within Groups	4556.23	69	66.03		
Psychological Domain	Pre Test	56.32	55.59	54.45	Between Groups	39.04	2	19.52	0.249	0.781
					Within Groups	5414.91	69	78.48		
	Post Test	57.72	65.37	60.05	Between Groups	798.70	2	399.35	3.259	**0.044**
					Within Groups	8456.29	69	122.56		
Social Domain	Pre Test	65.80	62.26	65.60	Between Groups	201.52	2	100.76	0.434	0.65
					Within Groups	16029.99	69	232.32		
	Post Test	74.28	78.04	67.50	Between Groups	1284.28	2	642.14	3.310	**0.042**
					Within Groups	13387.00	69	194.02		
Environmental Domain	Pre Test	73.20	73.30	70.80	Between Groups	86.82	2	43.41	0.459	0.634
					Within Groups	6526.83	69	94.59		
	Post Test	82.64	84.85	75.15	Between Groups	1141.39	2	570.70	3.341	**0.041**
					Within Groups	11785.72	69	170.81		

Data expressed in Mean, Sum of squares, Mean squares, F value and Statistical significance *(p< .044*, p< .042*, p< .041*);*df- degree of freedom, DYP- Diabetic Yoga Protocol

4.2.6 Comparison of the group wise differences among control 6 weeks and 12 weeks DYP group in domains of QoL:

Table 4.26 showing analysis of variances on various domains of QoL i.e. Physical, Psychological, Social and environmental between 6 weeks DYP group, 12 weeks DYP group and control group. The Physical domain for pre-test shows the mean scores of 56.96, 55.00 and 57.90 for 6 weeks DYP group, 12 weeks DYP group and control group respectively. The calculated F ratio 0.690 shows that physical domain at pre-test level was statistically insignificant (p=0.505) between groups. Similar results were obtained after post –test for physical domain, which shows non – significant (p=0.175) differences between groups with F ratio 1.785 as shown in Figure 4.20.

Additionally, psychological domain at pre-test shows no-significant differences between 6 weeks DYP (56.32) group, 12 weeks DYP (55.59) group and control group (54.45) with F ratio 0.249 (p=0.781). Though, at post-test for psychological domain statistically significant differences was seen between the groups (6 weeks DYP group-57.72, 12 weeks DYP group - 65.37 and control group-60.05) with F ratio 3.259 (p=0.044).

Furthermore, the mean scores of social domainfor6 weeks DYP group, 12 weeks DYP group and control group were 65.80, 62.26 and 65.60 respectively. The social domain pre-test calculated F ratio .434 was found to be statistically insignificant (p=0.650) between the groups. In contrast, significant differences was found between the groups on social domain for post-test with F ratio 3.310 (p =0. 042) as shown in figure 4.13.Moreover, environmental domain for pre-test for 6 weeks DYP group (73.2000), 12 weeks DYP group (73.2963) and control group shows no significant differences with F ratio of .459 (p= 0.634)

Although, the post-test for environmental domain shows statistically significant differences between the groups (6 weeks DYP group-82.64, 12 weeks DYP group- 84.85, control group- 75.15) with F ratio 3.341 with p= 0.041 as shown in Figure 4.20.

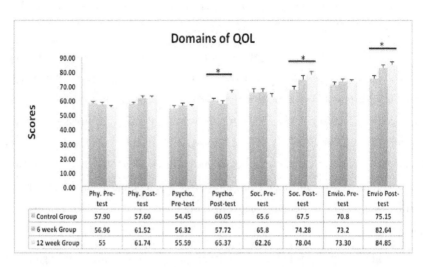

	Phy. Pre-test	Phy. Post-test	Psycho. Pre-test	Psycho. Post-test	Soc. Pre-test	Soc. Post-test	Envio. Pre-test	Envio Post-test
Control Group	57.90	57.60	54.45	60.05	65.6	67.5	70.8	75.15
6 week Group	56.96	61.52	56.32	57.72	65.8	74.28	73.2	82.64
12 week Group	55	61.74	55.59	65.37	62.26	78.04	73.30	84.85

Figure 4.20: Mean difference between domains of QoL for pre-test and post-test among control group , 6 weeks and 12 weeks DYP group. Significant differences on psychological , social and environmental domain *(p< .044*, p< .042*, p< .041*)* were found at follow up but no significant changes were found on physical domain among the groups. Phy –Physical; Psycho- Psychological; Socio-Social; Enviro-Environmental, df- degree of freedom, DYP- Diabetic Yoga Protocol

Table 4.27: Analysis of variance among control, 6 weeks DYP group and 12 weeks DYP group on Quality of Life in mean, sum of squares, mean squares and F ratio with p- values.

Variables		Group Mean			Source of Variance	Sum of Squares	df	Mean Squares	F-Value	P-Value
		6 weeks	12 weeks	Control Group						
QOL	Pre test	251.96	246.15	248.75	Between Groups	438.99	2	219.50	0.281	0.756
					Within Groups	53824.12	69	780.06		
	Post test	278.40	290.30	260.35	Between Groups	10315.14	2	5157.57	3.983	**0.023**
					Within Groups	89354.18	69	1294.99		

Data expressed in mean, sum of squares, mean squares, F value and statistical significance *(p<0.023*)*QoL- Quality of Life, df- degree of freedom, DYP- Diabetic Yoga Protocol

4.2.7 Comparison of the group wise differences among control 6 weeks and 12 weeks DYP group on overall QoL:

Table 4.27 showing analysis of variances on QoL between 6 weeks DYP group, 12-weeks DYP group and control group. The mean scores for overall QoL at Pre-test (6 weeks DYP=251.96, 12-weeks DYP=246.15 and control- 248.75 group) was statistically insignificant with F ratio 0.281(p=.756). However, the mean scores for post test in 6 weeks DYP group, 12-weeks DYP group and control group were 278.40, 290.30 and 260.35 respectively. The post-test scores for Quality of Life shows statistical significant difference between the groups with F ratio of 3.983 (p< 0.023) as shown in Figure 4.21.

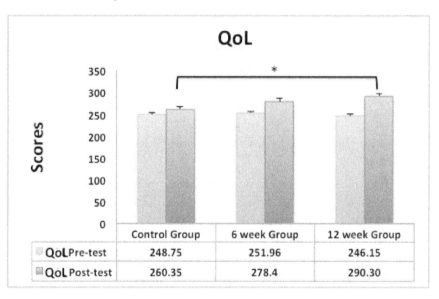

Figure 4.21: Mean difference between QoL for pre-test and post-test among Control group , 6 weeks and 12 weeks DYP group. Significant differences on QoL were seen at follow up among the groups (p< .023*).

Discussion of the results:

The comparison among the three defined groups for biochemical parameters i.e HbA1c and FBG shows no significant differences. Similar results were seen in Anthropometric parameters (Weight, BMI, HC, WHR), where no significant differences were observed among three groups except for WC (p=0.034). There was a significant difference between 12 weeks DYP and control group in WC (p=0.034).

However, no significant differences were found between Control and 6 weeks DYP and 6 weeks DYP group and 12 weeks DYP group.

Further, neuropsychological parameters like general health (p<0.001) and perceived stress (p=0.006) at post-test show significant differences among the three groups. The control group shows significant differences between both the DYP groups (6 weeks DYP & 12 weeks DYP) for general health and perceived stress. A significant improvement was observed in general health and perceived stress in both the DYP groups in comparison with control group. No significant differences were seen between both the DYP groups on general health and perceived stress. However, no significant differences were observed in sustained attention and state anxiety among three groups.

The molecular markers like Angiogenin (Pre-test (p<0.001) and post –test (p<0.001) and VEGF (Pre-test p= 0.005) shows significant differences among three groups. Among the groups, the significant differences were found in control group in comparison with both the DYP groups whereas no difference was found between the two DYP groups. The decline in mean values was seen in control group whereas increase in mean values was observed in both the DYP groups for angiogenesis. The neurogenesis marker i.e. BDNF shows no significant difference was seen among the three groups.

Furthermore, leptin shows significant differences between control and 12 weeks DYP group at pre-test level (p=0.027) but no post-test differences found among the groups Although, cortisol show no differences at both pre-test and post-test levels. Moreover, QoL (p=0.023) and its domains shows statistically significant differences at post-test level among three groups, but Physical domain shows no significant differences. The psychological domain shows significant difference between 6 weeks DYP and 12 weeks DYP group. 12 weeks DYP group shows significant improvement in psychological domain of QoL in comparison with 6 weeks DYP group. The Overall QoL, social and environmental domain shows significant improvement in 12W DYP group in comparison with the control group.

Among the DYP groups the maximum of the variables shown improvement in 12 weeks DYP group in comparison with control than 6 weeks DYP group. The results obtained from the present study supported the fact that longer duration of Yoga practices result in better homeostasis of the body. However, there are some variables, which didn't shown improvement in either of the groups which further suggest longer and adherent regime to be implemented in daily life.

128

Table 4.28: ANCOVA analysis for selected Biochemical (HbA1c, FBG), Anthropometric (weight, BMI, WC, HC and WHR) Neuropsychological (sustained attention, general health, state anxiety, perceived stress), Molecular (ANG, VEGF, BDNF), Hormonal (cortisol, leptin) and overall QoL in group mean, type III sum of squares , mean squares, F value with p values between control group and DYP group.

Variables	Group mean		Type III Sum of Squares	df	Mean Squares	F-Value	P-Value
	Control Group	DYP Group					
HbA1c	5.72	5.52	0.009	1	0.009	0.093	0.761
FBG	96.87	100.75	401.455	1	401.455	1.364	0.246
Weight	70.86	68.35	0.073	1	0.073	0.011	0.917
BMI	29.27	28.32	0.051	1	0.051	0.046	0.831
WC	97.50	91.54	268.275	1	268.275	6.763	**0.011**
HC	105.85	102.38	265.264	1	265.264	8.007	**0.006**
WHR	0.92	0.89	0.008	1	0.008	2.576	0.112
Sustained Attention	24.20	30.13	267.741	1	267.741	4.026	**0.049**
General Health	12.45	8.29	266.109	1	266.109	27.344	***< 0.001***
State Anxiety	36.60	31.83	551.287	1	551.287	9.369	**0.003**
Perceived Stress	17.26	13.26	387.438	1	387.438	12.695	**0.001**
Angiogenin	5.511	0.752	15.292	1	15.292	2.132	0.147
VEGF	0.0162	0.0157	0.001	1	0.001	9.646	**0.002**
BDNF	25.94	58.53	2605.832	1	2605.832	0.556	0.458
Cortisol	0.0013	0.0016	7.09E-06	1	7.09E-06	4.56	**0.035**
Leptin	0.00042	0.00029	1.14E-08	1	1.14E-08	0.202	0.654
Physical Domain	57.60	61.63	313.619	1	313.619	5.355	**0.024**
Psychological Domain	60.05	61.69	24.065	1	24.065	0.183	0.67
Social Domain	67.50	76.23	1256.318	1	1256.318	7.528	**0.008**
Environmental Domain	75.15	83.79	693.298	1	693.298	5.257	**0.025**
QoL	260.35	284.58	8362.829	1	8362.829	8.952	**0.004**

Table 4.28 :Data expressed in Mean, SD, and Statistical significance ($p< 0.011*$, $p< 0.006**$, $p< 0.049*$ $p< 0.001***$), $p< 0.003**$ $p< 0.001**$, $p< 0.002**$ $p< 0.035*$, $p< 0.024*$,$p< 0.008**$ $p< 0.025*$, $p< 0.004**$) HbA1c- Glycated Haemoglobin, FBG- Fasting Blood Glucose; BMI- Body Mass Index; WC-Waist Circumference, HC- Hip Circumference; WHR- Waist Hip Ratio ; SD= Standard Deviation; VEGF- Vascular Endothelial Growth; BDNF- Brain Derived Neurotropic Factor, QoL-Quality of Life DYP- Diabetic Yoga Protocol. The p value was calculated by ANCOVA with pre value of the respective variable and age as covariates.

Table 4.28 Indicates the results of ANCOVA between control group and 12 Weeks DYP group (experimental group). Various study variables were compared using ANCOVA whilst adjusting for pre values of respective variables in all the groups and age. The mean difference of Waist circumference [F=6.763, p=0.011], Hip circumference [F=8.007, p=0.006], Sustained attention [F=4.026, p=0.049], General health [F=27.344, p<0.001], State anxiety [F=9.369, p=0.003], Perceived stress [F=12.695, p=0.001], VEGF [F=9.646, p=0.002], Cortisol [F=4.560, p=0.035]], Physical domain [F=5.355, p=0.024], Social domain of QoL [F=7.528, p=0.008], Environmental domain of QoL [F=5.257, p=0.025] and QoL [F=8.952, p=0.004] were found significant while adjusting mean for age and pre values for all these respective variables. The mean difference of HbA1c [F= 0.093, p=0.761], FBG [F=1.364, p=0.246], weight [F=0.011, p=0.917], BMI [F=0.046, p=0.831], WHR [F= 2.576, p=0.112], Angiogenin [F=2.132, p=0.147], BDNF [F=0.556, p=0.458], leptin [F=0.202, p=0.654] and Psychological domain of QoL [F=0.183, p=0.670] were not found significant between these two groups

Table 4.29: ANCOVA analysis for selected Biochemical (HBA1c, FBG), Anthropometric (Weight, BMI, WC, HC and WHR) Neuropsychological (Sustained attention, General health, State anxiety, Perceived stress), Molecular (Angiogenin, VEGF, BDNF), Hormonal (Cortisol, Leptin) and overall QoL in Group mean, Type III sum of squares , Mean Squares, F value with p values among control group and 6 weeks DYP and 12 weeks DYP group.

Variables	Group Mean			Type III Sum of Squares	df	Mean Squares	F-Value	P-Value
	Control Group	6 weeks	12 weeks					
HbA1c	5.72	5.47	5.57	0.009	2	0.005	0.048	0.953
FBG	96.87	98.64	102.33	526.139	2	263.069	0.888	0.415
Weight	70.86	70.44	66.88	57.979	2	28.989	4.716	**0.011**
BMI	29.27	29.17	27.72	10.032	2	5.016	4.896	**0.009**
WC	97.51	91.73	91.40	268.808	2	134.404	3.354	**0.039**
HC	105.68	103.46	101.63	350.397	2	175.199	5.375	**0.006**
WHR	0.92	0.89	0.90	0.012	2	0.006	2.031	0.137
Sustained Attention	24.20	31.52	28.85	281.794	2	140.897	2.094	0.131
General Health	12.45	9.24	7.41	300.487	2	150.243	16.045	*< 0.001*
State Anxiety	36.6	32.52	31.19	568.61	2	284.305	4.781	**0.011**

Perceived Stress	17.26	13.61	13.02	408.523	2	204.262	6.672	**0.002**
Angiogenin	5.51	1.08	0.53	15.951	2	7.975	1.101	0.337
VEGF	0.016	0.015	0.016	0.001	2	0	4.798	**0.01**
BDNF	25.73	80.33	42.04	2660.081	2	1330.04	0.281	0.756
Cortisol	0.0012	0.0018	0.0015	7.20E-06	2	3.60E-06	2.294	0.106
Leptin	0.00042	0.00028	0.00030	1.45E-08	2	7.24E-09	0.127	0.881
Physical Domain	57.60	61.52	61.74	317.419	2	158.71	2.673	0.076
Psychological Domain	60.05	57.72	65.37	816.426	2	408.213	3.354	**0.041**
Social Domain	67.50	74.28	78.04	1647.652	2	823.826	5.038	**0.009**
Environmental Domain	75.15	82.64	84.85	863.299	2	431.65	3.287	**0.043**
QoL	260.35	278.4	290.30	11761.652	2	5880.826	6.553	**0.003**

Data Expressed in Mean, SD, and statistical significance (p< 0.011*, p< 0.009**, p< .0039* p< 0.006**, *p< 0.001****,p< 0.011*, p< 0.002** p< 0.010*, p< 0.041*,p< 0.009** p< 0.043*, p< 0.003**) HbA1c- GlycatedHaemoglobin, FBG-Fasting Blood Glucose; BMI- Body Mass Index; WC-Waist Circumference, HC- Hip Circumference; WHR- Waist Hip Ratio, SD= Standard Deviation; VEGF- Vascular Endothelial Growth; BDNF- Brain Derived Neurotropic Factor, QoL-Quality of Life DYP- Diabetic Yoga Protocol. The p value was calculated by ANCOVA with pre value of the respective variable and age as covariates. The p value was calculated by ANCOVA with pre value of the respective variable and age as covariates.

Table 4.29 Indicates the results of ANCOVA among control group, 6 weeks DYP group and 12 weeks DYP group (experimental groups). Various study variables were compared using ANCOVA whilst adjusting for pre values of respective variables in all the groups and age. The mean difference of weight [F=4.716, p=0.011], BMI [F=4.896, p=0.009], waist circumference [F=3.354, p=0.039], Hip circumference [F=5.375, p=0.006], General health [F=16.045, *p< 0.001]*, State anxiety [F=4.781, p=0.011], Perceived stress [F=6.672, p=0.002], VEGF [F=4.798, p=0.010], Psychological domain of QoL [F=3.354, p=0.041], Social domain of QoL [F=5.038, p=0.009], Environmental domain of QoL [F=3.287, p=0.043] and QoL [F=6.553, p=0.003] were found significant while adjusting mean for age and pre values for all these respective variables. The mean difference of HbA1c [F= 0.048, p=0.953], FBG [F=0.888, p=0.415], WHR [F= 2.031, p=0.137], Sustained attention [F=2.094, p=0.131], Angiogenin [F=1.101, p=0.337], BDNF [F=0.281, p=0.756],

Cortisol [F=2.294, p=0.106], Leptin [F=0.127, p=0.881] and Physical domain [F=2.673, p=0.076] were not found significant among these three groups.

Discussion of the results:

The Analysis of covariance (ANCOVA) was obtained by keeping pre scores as covariate and post scores as dependent variable. The comparison between control and DYP group was done while adjusting for age pre scores for the tested variable.

The WC, HC, sustained attention, general health, state anxiety, perceived stress, VEGF, cortisol, physical, social, environmental domains and overall QoL shows significant results in control and DYP group. On the other hand, comparison among three groups shows significant results on weight, BMI, WC, HC, general health, state anxiety, perceived stress, VEGF, Psychological, social, Environmental and overall QoL. However, the remaining variables didn't show significant results.

The promising result of DYP on the mentioned variables was observed. The variables, which didn't show significant results, may need further investigation for long term Yoga intervention that might bring positive and effective results on the insignificant parameters and also might help in maintenance of significant parameters.

4.3 Confronting the possible mechanism of Diabetic Yoga Protocol (DYP) induced effects on angiogenesis, neurogenesis, glycemic index, anthropometrical and neuropsychological factors in pre-diabetic pathophysiology:

The present study involved those participants in the study, which were found to at high risk after according to IDRS (≥60). IDRS was constructed by Mohan et al., (2005) and highlights the risk status of the individual in a most convenient way. It consists of 4 simple criteria i.e. Age, Level of physical activity, Waist circumference and parental history, which are considered to be the major risk factors for Diabetes. The present study is the first that explores the effect of DYP in angiogenesis, neurogenesis and on pro-inflammatory markers like cortisol and leptin respectively.

Various studies have focused upon the effect of Yogic practices on Diabetics and pre-diabetics. However, these studies mainly emphasize upon their glycemic, biochemical, and anthropometrical and neuropsychological profile of high-risk individuals. There are a few studies available that focused upon the neurogenesis and angiogenesis mechanisms in pre-diabetics. Moreover, the present study is unique in its way because it uses specific DYP, which designed specifically for pre-diabetic and for Diabetics. However, there are very little studies available, which focused upon the role of molecular survival in pre-diabetics.

A study has reported that by implementing healthy lifestyle changes and emphasizing on weight reduction one can curtail the risk of Diabetes by 58% in pre-diabetic stage (Lindstrom et al., 2006). Yoga can be an effective regime that mainly focuses upon the overall development of the individuals by emphasizing upon the healthy body and mind (Shiju et al., 2019). A study has shown beneficial role of Yoga in lessoning the possibility of developing Diabetes and its associated complications in people with pre-diabetes (Jyotsna, 2014). Several studies have highlighted the effectiveness of lifestyle modification tools in prevention and management of the Diabetes (Echouffo et al., 2012;Knowleret al., 2002; Tuomilehto et al., 2001 and Ramachandran et al., 2006). Furthermore, studies have also stated that Yogic practices curb the possibility of T2DM in adult population (Hegdeet al., 2013; McDermott et al., 2014 and Mooventhan, 2017).

In the present study, we examined the biochemical, molecular, anthropometric and psychological effects of DYP on pre-diabetic or high risk individuals in order to understand the impact of Yoga as a promising preventive regimen for pre-diabetic or high risk individuals.

Pre-diabetes is intermediatory state between normal glycaemia and hyperglycemia. In pre-diabetes, the glucose level begins to rise gradually along with onset of insulin resistance (earlier stage). The glycemic, anthropometric, neuropsychological parameters along with angiogenesis and neurogenesis play important role in pathology of Diabetes and pre-diabetes. There may be a link between the mentioned factors in the diseased conditions. These risk factors are possibly responsible for accumulation of Diabetes if not ameliorate at pre-diabetic stage via adopting healthy lifestyle (Yoga, physical exercise and diet) as shown Figure 4.22.

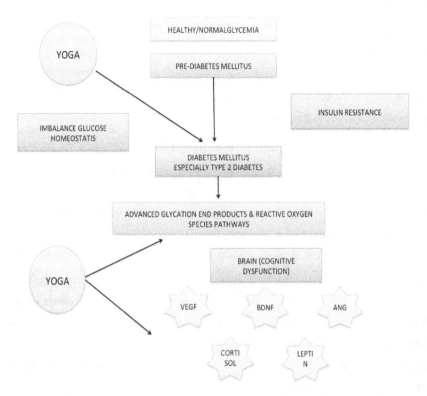

Figure 4.22: Schematic presentation of Yoga induced effects on homeostasis balance of the body. BDNF- Brain Derive Neurotropic Factor; ANG- Angiogenin ; VEGF-Vascular Endothelial Growth Factor.

It is well documented in the previous literature that Yoga is a rejuvenating therapy for Diabetes and pre-diabetes. In the present study we found out an associated link between Yoga and its effect on selected parameters and biomarkers.

The Yogic/physical activity increases the angiogenesis (VEGF and Angiogenin levels) (Park et al., 2010) and facilitates by blood and oxygen flow to the demanding parts of the body (exercised muscle) (Vital et al., 2014) by formation of new blood vessels. VEGF also broaden the artery diameter and expand the capillary network (Bloor, 2005). Yoga plays a potent role in activation of angiogenesis in the human physiology. In contrast the process of angiogenesis is altered in diseased (Prior et al., 2003) and unexercised condition. Moreover, decreased expression of VEGF in pancreatic β cells can hamper the effectiveness of insulin and consequently leads to the pre-diabetes in adults. Similarly, meta-analysis on effect of exercise on VEGF expression has been done in elderly persons. The results have demonstrated increased expression of VEGF in this population. Therefore, studies have suggested the stimulatory effect of exercise/Yoga on angiogenesis and its impact on overall well being. In Diabetic conditions, if there is an insufficient production of blood vessels then it may result into slow wound healing (Cheng and Xing, 2015).

The increased VEGF further triggers neurogenesis, thus VEGF act as meditator between angiogenesis and neurogenesis (Cao et al., 2004). Yoga and physical exercise increase the BDNF production, which (Luders et al., 2009 and Gotink et al., 2016) is a marker of neurogenesis. Neurogenesis helps in neuroplasticity and enhances hippocampal volume. BDNF brings positive changes in learning, memory, attention, cognitive functions, mental well being (Huang et al., 2014) and QoL. It further helps in eradicating depression, stress and anxiety of the individual via. Hippocampal activity .A possible mechanism for increase in BDNF levels is by increase in vagal tone (Brown and Gerbarg, 2005 and Khattab et al., 2007) by Yoga & meditation. BDNF increase by activation of parasympathetic nervous system via vagus nerve (Follesa et al., 2007).

The enhanced BDNF levels acts as a facilitator between brain well being and meditative practices (Cahn et al., 2017). A study reported increase in BDNF levels and its neuropsychological parameters after Yoga and combination of Yoga (Hallappa et al., 2018).

BDNF improves hippocampal plasticity, (Vivar et al., 2013) volume and it's functioning (Luders et al., 2009). Improved Hippocampal functioning help in better functioning of CAR (Fries et al., 2009) via HPA activity (stimulates through Yoga/exercise) and thus there is close relationship between BDNF and CAR (Cahn et al., 2017). The CAR is associated with increase in alertness, capacity to meet day-to-day demands and morning wakefulness (Fries et al., 2009 and Clow et al., 2010). The positive impact of Yoga and meditative practices also reported in the previous studies (Matousek et al., 2011). A Yogic and meditative practice helps in bringing the better quality of sleep, which further rejuvenates CAR functioning (Cahn et al., 2017).A negative correlation was found between stress and BDNF levels.(Schmidt and Duman, 2007). Thus, enhancement in BDNF result into declined stress whereas decline in BDNF level associated with increased stress.

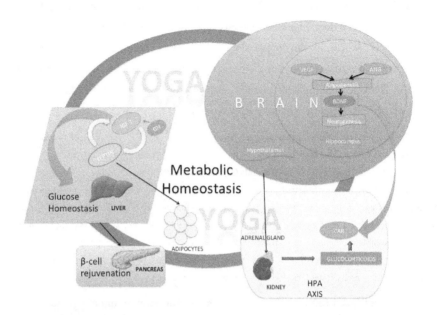

Figure 4.23:Schematic presentation of possible mechanism of action of Yoga on selected parameters and biomarkers; the possible interaction between Physical Exercise/Yoga with different genes and systems in the body. IGF-1 – Insulin Growth Factor-1; GH- Growth Hormone; BDNF- Brain Derive Neurotropic Factor; ANG-Angiogenin ; VEGF- Vascular Endothelial Growth Factor ; CAR- Cortisol Awakening Response; HPA- Hypothalmus Pitutary Adrenal; VEGF- Vascular Endothelial Growth Factor; BDNF – Brain Derived Neurotropic factor; ANG-Angiogenin; HPA- Axis – Hypothalamus–Pituitary-Adrenal Axis;IGF-1- Insulin Growth Factor-1; CAR- Cortisol Awakening Response

Moreover, Yoga/exercise and physical activity also increase the IGF-I (Raju and Nagendra) (Maass et al., 2016) signaling in brain, which correlates with insulin resistance (Friedrich et al.,2012) and associates with increased possibility of T2DM. Lower level of IGF-I level increases the insulin resistance and risk of Diabetes increases.

A study, (Uysal et al., 2017) has shown connectivity between IGF-1, and Leptin levels that helps in regulating the energy balance among body and brain. IGF-1 &Leptin regulate expression of each other (Li et al., 2005). Leptin act as moderator by activating IGF-1 gene in the liver and plays role in endocrinal growth (Won et al., 2016). Further IGF- 1 and leptin promote neurogenesis and hippocampal functionality and can cross the blood brain barrier (Reinhardt and Bondy, 1994), (Ahima et al., 1999). Leptin plays a dual role as it is expressed in both fat cells and CNS; it also controls the appetite along with brain development (Uysal et al., 2017). Both IGF-1 and leptin play the neuro-protective (Morrison, 2009 and Teryaeva, 2015) role in the brain. The increased leptin levels associates with obesity that result into leptin resistance (Tells et al., 2014). The possible reason of obesity is leptin resistance in which body is resistant to leptin and body do not responds to leptin signals of stop eating.

There may be an interconnection between different biomarkers and Yogic and meditative interventions. The Yogic and meditation interventions bring positive impact on VEGF, BDNF, Angiogenin, IGF-1, leptin, CAR and neuropsychological and anthropometric parameters as shown Figure 4.23.

The increased BDNF levels show positive impacts on neuropsychological parameters by improving mental and psychological well-being. The proper functioning of CAR activity is helpful in maintaining homeostasis in the body. Leptin plays the major role in maintaining neurocognitive functions along with regulation of appetite. Leptin is helpful in maintaining and controlling body weight.

Mental health is closely associated with progression of pre-diabetes to Diabetes. Depression and anxiety can two fold increase the risk of Diabetics at pre Diabetic level (Deschenes et al., 2016). There is evidence that show that aerobic exercise shows significant positive impact on psychological parameters on pre-Diabetes (Taheri et al., 2019).

The possible mechanism of action behind the efficacy of Yoga in T2D on Glycemic control might be enhanced sensitivity of b-cell in pancreas that help in better functioning of these pancreatic b-cells (Khatri et al., 2007). Yoga also improves BMI, weight, WC, HC and WHR by increasing the energy expenditure.

Hence, Yoga was found to be helpful in maintaining glucose control of the body and help in delay the conversion of pre-diabetes into Diabetes by actively working on the risk factors associated with it and plays a promising role in different possible mechanism of actions in the body, which might be the reason in developing the Diabetes in near future. So, Yoga/Physical activity balances the homeostasis of the body and maintains psychoneuroendocrine equilibrium as shown in Figure 4.23.

4.4   TESTING OF HYPOTHESIS

Hypothesis 01. Stated that "There would be significant effects of DYP practice on selected Biochemical variables i.e FBG and HbA1c among pre-diabetic women". The results of the present study revealed that pre & post scores for HbA1c was statistically significant at 0.05 level of significance whereas pre test & post test scores for FBG shows non-significant results at 0.05 level of significance. **Hence, the stated hypothesis was partially accepted.**

Hypothesis 02. Stated that "There would be significant effects of DYP practice on selected Anthropometric variables viz. body weight, BMI, WC, HC and Waist Hip Ratio (WHR) among pre-diabetic women". The results of the present study revealed that all the anthropometric variables (body weight, BMI, WC & HC) were statistically significant at 0.05 level of significance except WHR which were not significant at 0.05 level of significance. **Thus, the stated hypothesis was partially accepted.**

Hypothesis 03. Stated that "There would be significant effects of DYP practice on selected neuropsychological variables i.e state anxiety, perceived stress, sustained attention and general health among pre-diabetic women". The results of the present study revealed that all the neuropsychological parameters like attention, state anxiety, perceived stress and general health were statistically significant at 0.05 level of significance .**Thus, the stated hypothesis was accepted.**

Hypothesis 04. Stated that "There would be significant effects of DYP practice on selected molecular markers viz. Angiogenin, VEGF and BDNF among pre-diabetic women". The results of the present study revealed that pre & post scores for VEGF and Angiogenein was found to be statistically significant at 0.05 level of significance. However, pre & post scores for BDNF shows statistically non-significant results at 0.05 level of significance. **Accordingly, the stated hypothesis was partially accepted.**

Hypothesis 05. Stated that "There would be significant effects of DYP practice on selected Hormonal markers i.eLeptin and cortisol among pre-diabetic women". The results of the present study revealed that Pre & post scores for cortisol was found to

138

be statistically significant at 0.05 level of significance whereas Leptin shows no statistical significant difference at pre & post scores at 0.05 level of significance. **So,the stated hypothesis was partially accepted.**

Hypothesis 06. Stated "There would be significant effects of DYP practice on total Quality of life (QoL) and its domains among pre-diabetic women". The results of the present study revealed that pre & post scores was found to be statistically significant at 0.01 level of significance. **Thus, the stated hypothesis was accepted.**

Hypothesis 07. Stated that "There would be significant effects of practicing DYP for 6 weeks and 12 weeks on selected Biochemical variables viz. FBG and HbA1c among pre-diabetic women" .The results of the present study revealed that pre & post scores for HbA1c and FBG was statistically significant at 0.05 level of significance in 6W DYP group whereas in 12W DYP group pre test & post test scores for HbA1c and FBG shows statistically non-significant difference. **Hence, the stated hypothesis was partially accepted.**

Hypothesis 08. Stated that "There would be significant effects of practicing DYP for 6 weeks and 12 weeks on selected Anthropometric variables i.e body weight, BMI, WC, HC and WHR among pre-diabetic women". The results of the present study revealed that Pre & Post scores for all the selected anthropometric parameters shows statistically non significant results in 6W DYP group. However, in 12W DYP group all the anthropometric variables (body weight, BMI, WC & HC) were statistically significant at 0.05 level of significance except Waist-Hip Ratio which was found to be statistically non-significant. **Hence, the stated hypothesis was partially accepted.**

Hypothesis 09. Stated that "There would be significant effects of practicing DYP for 6 weeks and 12 weeks on selected Neuro-psychological variables i.e state anxiety, perceived stress, sustained attention and general health among pre-diabetic women". The results of the present study revealed that pre & post scores was found to be statistically significant at 0.01 level of significance in both the groups i.e 6W DYP and 12W DYP group .**Thus, the stated hypothesis was accepted.**

Hypothesis 10. Stated that "There would be significant effects of practicing DYP for 6 weeks and 12 weeks on molecular markers viz. Angiogenin,VEGF and BDNF among pre-diabetic women".The results of the present study revealed that pre & post scores for selected molecular markers shows statistically non- significant results in both the groups i.e 6W DYP group and 12W DYP group except Angiogenin which shows statistically significant results at 0.05 level of significance in 6W DYP group . **Thus, the stated hypothesis was partially accepted.**

Hypothesis 11. Stated that "There would be significant effects of practicing DYP for 6 weeks and 12 weeks on hormonal markers *i.e*leptin and cortisol among pre-diabetic women". The results of the present study revealed that pre & post scores for leptin and cortisol was found to be statistically non-significant at 0.05 level of significance in 6W DYP and 12W DYP group. **Hence, the stated hypothesis was rejected.**

Hypothesis 12. Stated that "There would be significant effects of practicing DYP for 6 weeks and 12 weeks on total QoL and its associated domains among pre-diabetic women". The results of the present study revealed that pre & post scores was found to be statistically significant at 0.05 level of significance for total QoL and its associated domains in both the 6W DYP and 12W DYP groups except psychological domain which shows statistically non-significant results in 6W DYP group..**Thus, the stated hypothesis was accepted.**

CHAPTER – V
SUMMARY, FINDINGS, CONCLUSIONS AND
RECOMMENDATIONS

5.1   SUMMARY OF THE PRESENT STUDY

"The sooner people find out that they have pre-diabetes and take action, the better are their chances of preventing type 2 diabetes".

-    **Ann Albright, PhD, RD**
Director, Division of   Diabetes   Translation

Diabetes Mellitus (DM) is a metabolic disorder associated with alteration in the carbohydrate metabolism leading to increased blood sugar level called hyperglycemia. The condition may arise due to decreased insulin secretion (Type 1 Diabetes Mellitus (T1DM)), or altered action of insulin (Type 2 Diabetes Mellitus (T2DM)). Previous studies suggest that risk of DM increases with the increase in age, sedentary lifestyle, obesity and imbalance in energy intake (Pal et al., 2017). Several organizations working at national or international level to control the DM and some of the renowned organizations includes World Health Organization (WHO), American Diabetes Association (ADA), International Diabetes Federation (IDF), World Diabetes Foundation (WDF), and India Diabetes Research Foundation (IDRF). India is fast becoming the Diabetic capital. The increase in the number of incidents hampers the progression of any developing nation and increases the economical burden on the government. A slight positive change in our daily life style may reduce the risk of developing Diabetes or the progression can be halted at initial stages if one gets to know his/her status. Therefore, controlling the transition of pre-diabetes to Diabetes is important.

Yoga is mind-body interaction technique and is being practiced worldwide. The positive impact of Yoga has led the world to celebrate International Yoga Day on 21st June. Archeological evidences suggest that Yoga begin in India around 3000 B.C (Sengupta, 2012). Yoga is popularly known to be a mind-body interaction technique based on a set of physical exercises called *asanas* and breathing exercises called *pranayama* (Sengupta, 2012). In view of this Ministry of AYUSH, Government of India has developed a specific set of Yoga protocol called Diabetic Yoga Protocol

(DYP). The protocol comprises of a set of loosening exercises, *asanas*, *pranayama*, *suryanamaskara*, and meditation (Nagarathna et al., 2019). Although there are many studies assessing the benefits of Yoga in Diabetes, but major limitation is the lack of specific protocol and also the mechanism involved is poorly understood. Hence, we attempted to analyze the effectiveness of DYP by means of both biochemical and molecular profiling of pre-diabetic women.

The present study focused upon the preventive approach for amelioration and timely management of Diabetes or pre-diabetes. The pre-diabetic stage remains undetected in the community due to the lack of awareness or ignoring preliminary symptoms. The present study focused upon to check the risk status for Diabetes by using simple and economical tool called Indian Diabetes Risk Score (IDRS) developed by Mohan et al. (2005) among the community. Moreover, by knowing the risk status for the Diabetes a person can adopt preventive measures to delay or stop the conversion from pre-diabetes to Diabetes.

There are a multiple studies available which shows the beneficial effects of Yoga and physical activity on inhibiting the progression towards Diabetes. (Rammoorthi et al., 2019; Keerthi et al., 2017; Yang et al., 2011 and Ramchandran et al., 2006)

Yoga is a combination of physical postures, breathing exercises and meditative practices, which focused upon the wholesome (Physical, mental & emotional) development of the individual (Nayak and Shankar, 2004 and Yang et al., 2011). There are various risk factors (obesity, family history, level of physical activity, abdominal obesity), which contribute in progression from pre-diabetes and Diabetes, and Yoga is an influential way in curbing these risk factors. A candidate gene also plays major role in pathophysiology of Diabetes or pre-diabetes. This is the first study, which attempts to explore the molecular effect of specific DYP proposed by Ministry of AYUSH.

The present work is experimental nature and it is focused upon 3 months effects of Diabetic Yoga Protocol in molecular, biochemical, neuropsychological and anthropometrical profile of Pre Diabetic women. The individuals with IDRS $\geq$60 was recruited in the present study after informed consent obtained from participants and then divided into control and Yoga Groups.

After exclusion of dropouts from the present study the remaining number found to be N=34 (Control Group) and N= 68 (DYP Group). The DYP group further divided into 6 weeks DYP Group (N=28) and 12 weeks DYP Group (N= 40) based on their presence and absence in the Yoga classes. The selected parameters like biochemical (HbA1c, FBG), molecular (angiogenin, VEGF, BDNF, cortisol, leptin), anthropometric (weight, BMI, WC, HC, WHR) and neuropsychological (sustained attention, perceived stress, state anxiety, general health) and overallQoL were measured at baseline (pre-test) and after 3 months (post-test).

5.2   FINDINGS OF THE STUDY

Based on objectives, hypothesis, and limitation of the present study the following findings was obtained:

1.   **Effect of pre- post analysis on selected biochemical parameters i.e HbA1c and FBG in control and DYP group.**

The result for Pre-Post analysis for biochemical parameters (HbA1c and FBG) (Table 4.1)shows that HBA1c reported significant changes after pre-post analysis in DYP group (p=0.004) and control Group (p=0.024) whereas FBG shows non-significant changes in DYP as well as Control group.

2.   **Effect of pre-post analysis on selected anthropometric parameters like weight, BMI, WC, HC and WHR in control and DYP group.**

The result of the present study revealed that all the anthropometric parameters(Table 4.2) like Weight (p=0.005), BMI (p=0.016), WC (p=0.019) and HC (p=0.024) shows significant decline after pre-post analysis in DYP Group except WHR that shows non-significant results. In contrast, control group demonstrated non-significant results on all the selected anthropometric parameters in pre-post analysis (Table 4.3).

3.   **Effect of pre-post analysis on selected neuropsychological parameters namely sustained attention, state anxiety, perceived stress and general health in control and DYP group.**

Further, all the neuropsychological parameters(Table 4.4) viz. sustained attention (p<0.001), state anxiety (p<0.001), perceived stress (p<0.001), and general health (p<0.001), shows significant improvements in DYP group. However, in control

143

group, all the anthropometric parameters(Table 4.5) shows non-significant differences except state anxiety (p=0.015) which shows significant differences between pre-test and post-test analysis.

4. **Effect of pre-post analysis on selected molecular markers viz. angiogenin, VEGF and BDNF in control and DYP group.**

The angiogenesis markers like angiogenin (p=0.029) and VEGF (p=0.046) shown significant improvements in DYP group after pre-post analysis **(Table 4.6)**. The BDNF shows non-significant changes in pre-post analysis in DYP group. In control group, decline in markers of angiogenesis and neurogenesis **(Table 4.7)** was seen but significant decline on VEGF concentrations (p< 0.001) were seen after pre-post analysis.

5. **Effect of pre-post analysis on selected hormonal markers like cortisol and leptin in control and DYP group.**

The hormonal markers **(Table 4.8)** like cortisol (p=0.024) show significant differences whereas leptin shows no significant changes in DYP group after Pre-Post analysis. Both cortisol and leptin demonstrated non-significant changes in control group after pre-post analysis **(Table 4.8)**.

6. **Effect of Pre- Post analysis on total QoL and its associated domains like physical, psychological, social and environmental domain in control and DYP group.**

The domains of QoL (physical (p< 0.001), psychological (p< 0.001), social (p< 0.001), environmental (p< 0.001) and overall QoL (p< 0.001) **(Table 4.9)** show statistical significant improvements in DYP Group whereas in control group overall QoL (p=0.030) also improved significantly after Pre-post analysis, But, in control group **(Table 4.10)** none of the domains of QoL shows significant changes except psychological domain (p=0.031) which shows significant differences after Pre-Post analysis.

7. **Effect of pre-post analysis on selected Biochemical parameters i.e HbA1c and FBG in 6 weeks DYP Group and 12 weeks DYP group.**

In the present study the DYP group was further divided into 6 weeks DYP and 12 weeks DYP group according to presence in the Yoga class of the participants. The

6 weeks DYP group shows significant differences (Table 4.11) on both selected biochemical parameters i.e. HbA1c (p= 0.022) and FBG (p=0.038) at pre-post analysis. In contrast, no significant changes were reported after Pre-Post analysis in 12 weeks DYP group on selected biochemical parameters. (Table 4.11)

8. **Effect of pre-post analysis on selected anthropometric parameters like weight, BMI, WC, HC and WHR in 6 weeks DYP Group and 12 weeks DYP group.**

No significant changes were seen in any of the selected Anthropometric parameters(Table 4.12) after pre-post analysis in 6 weeks DYP group. However, significant improvements (Table 4.13) were seen in all the Anthropometric parameters i.e. weight (p< 0.001), BMI (p< 0.001), WC (p= 0.041) and HC (p= 0.018) except WHR in 12 weeks DYP group.

9. **Effect of pre-post analysis on selected neuropsychological parameters namely sustained attention, state anxiety, perceived stress and general health in 6 weeks DYP Group and 12 weeks DYP group.**

All the selected neuropsychological parameters like sustained attention (p< 0.001), state anxiety (p< 0.001), perceived stress (p< 0.001), and general health (p< 0.001) shown significant improvements in 6 weeks DYP Group after pre-post analysis (Table 4.14). Similarly, in 12 weeks DYP group significant improvements were seen on sustained attention (p=0.003), state anxiety (p< 0.001), perceived stress (p< 0.001), and general health (p< 0.001) (Table 4.15).

10. **Effect of pre-post analysis on selected molecular markers viz. angiogenin, VEGFand BDNF in 6 weeks DYP Group and 12 weeks DYP group.**

The molecular markers like angiogenin, VEGF and BDNF didn't reported any significant changes in both 6 weeks DYP (Table 4.16) and 12 weeks DYP (Table 4.17) group except angiogenin, which was significantly (p= .039) increased in 6 weeks DYP group after Pre-Post analysis.

11. **Effect of pre-post analysis on selected Hormonal markers like cortisol and leptin in 6 weeks DYP Group and 12 weeks DYP group.**

The selected hormonal markers like cortisol and leptin (Table 4.18) levels didn't show significant changes in 6 weeks DYP group and 12 weeks DYP group after pre-post analysis.

145

12. **Effect of pre-post analysis on overallQoL and its associated domains like physical, psychological, social and environmental domain in 6 weeks DYP Group and 12 weeks DYP group.**

It has been also found in the present study that all the domains of QoL and overall QoL shown significant improvements in 6 weeks DYP (physical-p=0.030, social-p=0.001, environmental-p=0.001, QoL-(p<0.001) (Table 4.19) and 12 weeks DYP group (physical-p=0.005, psychological- p<0.001, social-p<0.001, Environmental-(p<0.001), QoL- (p<0.001)(Table 4.20) except psychological domain which didn't show significant changes in 6 weeks DYP group at pre-post test level.

13. **Effect of group wise comparison (control and 6 weeks DYP Group & 12 weeks DYP group) in selected biochemical parameters i.e HbA1c and FBG.**

The results of the comparison among control, 6 weeks DYP and 12 weeks DYP group on biochemical parameters **(Table 4.21)** at pre test and post test shows non-significant results on the mentioned groups. However, alterations in biochemical parameters were seen among these groups.

14. **Effect of group wise comparison (Control and 6 weeks DYP Group & 12 weeks DYP group) in selected anthropometric parameters like weight, BMI, WC and HC and WHR.**

Anthropometric parameters (Table 4.22) didn't shows significant differences among the groups except waist circumference which shows statistical significant difference (p=0.034) between the 12 week DYP versus control group. No significant changes were seen in Control versus 6 weeks DYP group and 12 weeks DYP group and 6 weeks DYP group on waist circumference. However, the beneficial effects of DYP on anthropometric parameters were seen in both the intervention groups (6 weeks DYP Group and 12 weeks DYP group) but not at a significant level.

15. **Effect of group wise comparison (control and 6 weeks DYP Group & 12 weeks DYP group) in selected neuropsychological parameters namely sustained attention, state anxiety, perceived stress and general health.**

Neuropsychological parameters (Table 4.23) shown diverse results where statistically significant results were seen in general Health (p=< 0.001) and perceived

146

stress (p=0.006) but sustained attention & state anxiety shows non-significant differences among the mentioned groups after 3 months. The statistical significant difference on general health and perceived stress was found in Control versus 6 weeksDYP group and control versus 12 weeks DYP group. However, no significant differences were found between 6 weeks DYP group and 12 weeks DYP group. The improvements in selected neuropsychological parameters were seen in both the DYP groups in comparison with the control group.

16. **Effect of group wise comparison (control and 6 weeks DYP Group & 12 weeks DYP group) in selected molecular markers viz. angiogenin, VEGF and BDNF.**

The marker of angiogenesis like angiogenin (Table 4.24) shows significant differences(p<0.001) in control versus 6 weeksDYP group and control versus 12 weeks DYP group. However no significant differences were found between 6 weeks DYP and 12 weeks DYP group. Though, the significant improvements were seen in 6 weeks DYP and 12 weeks DYP in comparison with control group. Moreover, no significant differences were found among mentioned groups on VEGF and BDNF after 3 months. The 6 weeks DYP group and 12 weeks DYP group shows improvements in VEGF and BDNF levels in comparison with the control group but not at a significant level.

17. **Effect of group wise comparison (control and 6 weeks DYP Group & 12 weeks DYP group) in selected Hormonal markers like cortisol and leptin**

The cortisol and leptin level (Table 4.25) shows no significant differencesamong the mentioned groups. However, the baseline significant differences were found on leptin level (p< 0.027)among the groups.

18. **Effect of group wise comparison (control and 6 weeks DYP Group & 12 weeks DYP group) on overall QoL and its associated domains like physical, psychological, social and environmental domain**

The domains of QoL (Table 4.26) reported the statistically significant differences among the mentioned groups excluding Physical domain, which shows non-significant results. The psychological domain (p<0.044) shows significant difference between 6 weeks DYP group versus 12 weeks DYP group whereas social (p< 0.042)and environmental (p< 0.041) domain reported significant difference between Control and 6 weeks DYP group after 3 months. Furthermore, overall QoL

147

(Table 4.27) shows significant differences in control versus 12 weeks DYP group (p<0.023) but no significant differences found in 6 weeks DYP versus 12 weeks DYP and control versus 6 weeks DYP Group.

5.3   CONCLUSIONS

The findings of the present study bring to the following conclusions:

1. We have examined the effect of 3 months DYP practice on biochemical parameters and found that HbA1c significantly improved but no significant changes were observed in FBG. Similar result seen in control group where significant changes were seen in HbA1c and FBG reported no significant differences. The result of the present study supported the favorable impact of DYP on HbA1c, which is a most reliable method to check the glycemic status of the individual. The DYP help in maintaining the normalglycemia in the participants.

2. The significant impact of 3 months DYP practice was seen on body weight, BMI, WC and HC after pre-post analysis. The significant improvements were reported in all the selected anthropometric parameters in DYP group except WHR. However, control group shows no changes in anthropometric parameters at pre-post analysis. The result of the present study revealed the beneficial impact of DYP on anthropometric parameters.

3. The significant improvement of 3 months DYP practices shown on neuropsychological parameters like sustained attention, general health, state anxiety and perceived stress. In contrast, no significant changes were seen in control group on neuropsychological parameters except state anxiety. The result of the present study shows DYP as a potent way in improving the stress, anxiety and cognitive improvements in the pre-diabetic women. Stress is also one of the risk factor in Diabetes, which Yoga ameliorates. Thus, it reduces the risk for developing Diabetes.

4. The beneficial impact of 3 months DYP practice of Yoga was seen on markers of angiogenesis and neurogenesis. The angiogenin and VEGF levels show significant improvement but no significant changes were seen on BDNF. However the increase in mean levels was observed in BDNF levels. Later,

148

control group shows significant decline on angiogenin levels whereas non-significant changes were observed in VEGF and BDNF levels. However, decline in VEGF and BDNF were seen in control group. The result of our present study supports the role of Yoga in angiogenesis and neuronal survival.

5.   The hormonal markers like cortisol shows significant changes in DYP group whereas leptin shows insignificant results in DYP group. On the other hand, both cortisol and leptin shows no significant changes in control group. The result suggests that it might be possible that a longer duration of Yoga practices bring changes in the hormonal markers.

6.   It is also found in present study that domains of QoL and overall QoL significantly improved whereas in control group the significant improvement was seen only in psychological domain and overallQoL. In present study it was reported that DYP shows beneficial effect on QoL and its associated domains.

7.   The 6 weeks DYP group and 12 weeks DYP group shows the maintenance of normalglycemia   in the pre-diabetic participants according to HbA1c. However, 6 weeks DYP group shows significant changes on biochemical parameters in comparison with 12 weeks DYP Group

8.   The significant impacts of Yogic practices were seen 12 weeks DYP group in body weight, BMI, WC and HC whereas WHR didn't show significant differences after pre-post analysis. However, in 6 weeks DYP Group no significant changes were seen on anthropometric parameters. The present study shows that long term Yogic practices helps in improving anthropometric parameters.

9.   The neuropsychological parameters like sustained attention, state anxiety, perceived stress and general health shown significant improvements in 12 weeks DYP and 6 weeks DYP group after Yogic practices. The Yogic practices shows promising results on neuropsychological and cognitive parameters.

10. The angiogenin, VEGF and BDNF shows increase in 12 weeks DYP group after Yoga practices but not at significant level. The similar results were seen

149

in 6 weeks DYP group except angiogenin, which shows significant improvement after Yogic practices. The result shows the beneficial role of Yoga on angiogenesis and neurogenesis.

11.   The result of the present study demonstrated that no significant differences was found on hormonal makers (cortisol and Leptin) in both the intervention groups i.e 6 weeks DYP group and 12 weeks DYP group after 3 months of Yogic practices. The results of the present study suggest that it might be possible that long term of Yoga practice brings changes in hormonal markers.

12.   The significant impact of Yogic practices were seen in 6 weeks DYP group on domains of Quality of life like physical, social, environmental domain and overall QoL. However, the mean improvements were seen in psychological domain but not at significant level.

13.   The result of the present study demonstrated significant increase on all the domains of QoL (physical, psychological, social and environmental) and total QoL in 12 weeks DYP group after Yogic practices. The present study concluded that Yoga is helpful in improving QoL in the participants.

14.   The group wise comparison among control, 6 weeks DYP and 12 weeks DYP group shows significant differences of 12 weeks intervention on WC, general health, perceived stress, angiogenin, psychological domain, social domain, environmental domain of QoL and total QoL. The WC demonstrated significant changes in 12 week DYP in comparison with control group. Both the intervention groups i.e 6 weeks DYP and 12 weeks DYP group shows significant improvements on general health and perceived stress in control group. The angiogenin levels reported significant differences in control versus 6 weeks DYP group and control versus 12 weeks DYP group. Moreover, psychological domain, social domain, environmental domain and QoLshows significant differences in control versus 12 weeks DYP group. Though, psychological domain demonstrated significant difference in 6 weeks DYP group versus 12 weeks DYP group. The result of the present study revealed that long-term Yogic practice brings beneficial results on most of the parameters in comparison with control and 6 weeks DYP group. No significant differences were found in HbA1c, FBG, weight, BMI, HC, WHR,

sustained attention, state anxiety, VEGF, BDNF, cortisol, leptin and physical domain of QoL among the groups.

CPSIA information can be obtained
at www.ICGtesting.com
Printed in the USA
LVHW080524101222
734929LV00013B/552

9 789146 698067